Psychotherapeutic Treat
of Psychosis

This book explores the psychoanalytic treatment of a patient with psychosis from a range of different psychotherapeutic perspectives.

The psychotherapeutic treatment of psychotic individuals is both rare and controversial with a limitation in availability of clinical material. As psychoanalytically oriented therapy is private, it is almost impossible to "witness" the actual human interaction of therapeutic process. While catatonia is a rare disorder, there are many attempts to hypothesize a theoretical psychic structure for the range of disorders called psychotic. Therapists rarely report "successful" outcomes of long and unusual treatments. In the book, a fragment of the treatment of a catatonic adolescent is reconstructed as an endeavor in representing that which is not clinically representable. Following the case report, which also reveals part of the history of the therapist, prominent analytic clinicians of different theoretical orientations share their understanding and comment on the material revealed.

With a fresh perspective on psychoanalytic treatment of psychosis, this book is essential reading for psychoanalysts, psychotherapists, and clinicians involved in the treatment of psychosis.

Bennett E. Roth received a Ph.D. degree from New York University and then trained in both psychoanalysis and group therapy. He has contributed to journals in both fields with particular interest in difficult patients. Following consulting work after 9/11, he researched group violence that resulted in *A Group Analytic Approach to Mass Violence*.

Routledge Focus on Mental Health

Routledge Focus on Mental Health presents short books on current topics, linking in with cutting-edge research and practice.

Titles in the series:

Life Skills and Adolescent Mental Health
Can Kids Be Taught to Master Life?
Ole Jacob Madsen

Gender, Sexuality and Subjectivity
A Lacanian Perspective on Identity, Language and Queer Theory
Duane Rousselle

Lacan, Jouissance and the Social Sciences
The One and the Many
Raul Moncayo

Understanding and Coping with Illness Anxiety
Phil Lane

The Linguistic Turn of the English Renaissance
A Lacanian Perspective
Shirley Zisser

Psychotherapeutic Treatment of Psychosis
A Case of Catatonia and Discussion
Edited by Bennett E. Roth

For a full list of titles in this series, please visit
www.routledge.com/Routledge-Focus-on-Mental-Health/book-series/RFMH

Psychotherapeutic Treatment of Psychosis

A Case of Catatonia and Discussion

Edited by Bennett E. Roth

Routledge
Taylor & Francis Group

LONDON AND NEW YORK

First published 2024
by Routledge
4 Park Square, Milton Park, Abingdon, Oxon OX14 4RN

and by Routledge
605 Third Avenue, New York, NY 10158

Routledge is an imprint of the Taylor & Francis Group, an informa business

© 2024 selection and editorial matter, Bennett E. Roth; individual chapters, the contributors

The right of Bennett E. Roth to be identified as the author of the editorial material, and of the authors for their individual chapters, has been asserted in accordance with sections 77 and 78 of the Copyright, Designs and Patents Act 1988.

British Library Cataloguing-in-Publication Data
A catalogue record for this book is available from the British Library

ISBN: 978-1-032-70249-0 (hbk)
ISBN: 978-1-032-71386-1 (pbk)
ISBN: 978-1-003-42704-9 (ebk)

DOI: 10.4324/9781003427049

Typeset in Times New Roman
by Apex CoVantage, LLC

Contents

Contributors

Anthony Bass, Ph.D., is an associate professor and clinical consultant at the New York University Postdoctoral Program for Psychoanalysis and Psychotherapy. He is a faculty and training and supervising analyst at the Columbia University Center for Psychoanalytic Training and Research, in the Department of Psychiatry. He is a founder and the president of the Stephen Mitchell Relational Study Center, and a founding director of the International Association for Relational Psychoanalysis and Psychotherapy. He was a founding editor and editor emeritus of *Psychoanalytic Dialogues: the International Journal of Relational Perspectives*.

Priscilla F. Kauff, Ph.D., is Clinical Professor of Psychology in Psychiatry at Weill Medical College, Cornell University, where she teaches and supervises in the psychiatric residency and the psychology fellowship programs. She is also Distinguished Fellow of the American Group Psychotherapy Association and a member of the Editorial Board of the *International Journal of Group Psychotherapy*. Dr. Kauff maintains a private practice in New York City.

Eric R. Marcus, MD, is Professor of Clinical Psychiatry at Columbia University College of Physicians and Surgeons, and also Supervising and Training Psychoanalyst at Columbia University Center for Psychoanalytic Training and Research.

Annie Reiner, Ph.D., is a senior faculty member and training analyst at The Psychoanalytic Center of California (PCC) in Los Angeles. Her work was greatly influenced by Wilfred Bion, with whom she studied in the 1970s. She lectures throughout the world. She has published in numerous journals and anthologies and is the author of three psychoanalytic books, including *The Quest for Conscience: The Birth of the Mind* (Karnac, 2009), *Bion and Being: Passion and the Creative Mind* (Karnac, 2012), and *W. R. Bion's Theories of Mind: A Contemporary Introduction* (Routledge, 2022). She is also Editor of *Of Things Invisible to Mortal Sight: Celebrating the Work of James S. Grotstein* (Karnac, 2017). Dr. Reiner is also a poet, painter, and singer, and in addition to her psychoanalytic writings, she is the author of a book of short stories, four books of poems, and six children's books which she also illustrated. She supervises and maintains a psychoanalytic practice in Beverly Hills, California.

Bennett E. Roth, Ph.D., is formerly a training analyst in the International Psychoanalytical Association. He is the coauthor of the American Group Psychotherapy organization Monograph of *The Difficult Patient in Group* (International Universities Press, 1990) and the author of *The Group Analytic Approach to Understanding Mass Violence* (Routledge, 2018). He is Adjunct Assistant Professor in Mt. Sinai Department of Psychiatry and a frequent journal contributor. He is in private practice in New York City.

Karyn Todes, Ph.D., is a training psychoanalyst and a clinical and counseling psychologist in private practice in Sydney, Australia. She is a member of the Australian Psychoanalytic Society (APAS), the International Psychoanalytic Association (IPA), and the Australian Psychological Society (APS). Karyn was former National Scientific Chair of APAS, a former member on APAS's Executive Committee, and former Scientific Chair of the Sydney Branch. She is a committee member on the IPA Climate Committee and the IPA Scientific Committee. Her interests are especially focused on the exploration of psychotic processes and severe disturbance. Karyn is currently working on a chapter for a new book on psychoanalysis and climate change, and she is also coauthoring a chapter on psychoanalysis and climate change in the new edition of the *Textbook of Psychoanalysis*.

Paul Williams trained as a psychoanalyst with The British Psychoanalytical Society, where he was a training and supervising analyst. From 2001 to 2007, he was Joint Editor-in-Chief, with Glen Gabbard, of the *International Journal of Psychoanalysis* and Consultant Psychotherapist in the National Health Service in Belfast, Northern Ireland, where he treated traumatized patients. He now lives and works in private psychoanalytic practice in Northern California. He has published many papers and books on the subject of severe disturbance and psychosis. Recently, he produced an experimental literary trilogy on psychosis as seen from the inside: *The Fifth Principle* (Routledge, 2010), *Scum* (Routledge, 2013), and *The Authority of Tenderness* (Routledge, 2021).

Introduction

Bennett E. Roth

Documentarians create nonfiction films to present *a cinematic narrative* using various techniques and compelling story structures to arouse audiences to care about the subject matter on the screen. I hope that I have achieved a portion of that with the "story of a catatonic boy." The usual case-study format did not seem appropriate for this effort. Rather than presenting my "understanding" of a case that could cast me as knowledgeable, I presented an early clinical effort to stimulate a search to understand the possible dynamics in that event. I experimented with the usual case-study approach to engage readers' creative freedom to clinically understand and interpret and possibly to learn (Coen, 2000). Any reader is then free to creatively engage with the actual material, to use it as they need to, and to learn from my experience to understand the event or to enhance their analytic understanding. What followed is a surprisingly wide understanding of that dynamic encounter. One benefit of this approach is that every respondent had access to the same material revealing an incredibly wide and evocative range of understanding of psychotherapeutic events and process with a critically disturbed boy. Not to be ignored are those who choose not to respond to my invitation to participate.

I think a wider theoretical understanding that encounter is necessary. Adolescence is a time during which children acquire the social and cognitive skills they will need as adults. Just as critically, it is also the time in which their brains develop – or fail to develop – in a way that enables them to create their full potential or become the prerequisites for psychopathological conflicts. Research findings reveal that signs of emotional and cognitive deficits appear developmentally earlier, while the thrust of movement from within the family to social interaction and independence is often a significant factor in terms of revealing developmental deficits. Human motivational/emotional systems play a crucial role in emerging social relationships and in contained mental functioning. *Inter-male* aggression, also aptly called *dominance motivational/ emotional system*, is that which regulates social interactions between nearly sexually matured adolescents. The irregular pattern of maturation of these motivational/emotional systems requires their sporadic integration with the phylogenetically more recent Attachment/CARE Systems that primarily

DOI: 10.4324/9781003427049-1

governed the subject's relationships until puberty. The neurobiological goal is our complex human capacity to safely share a multiplicity of self-states that includes activity, sensations, emotions, thinking, as well as a variety of safe attachments and separations.

In addition to the above, these interactive systems act in complementary connection with FEAR/threat motivational/emotional system that regulates submissive behavior and (fear of) social defeat. The fear-defense system is an evolutionarily innate system organizing hard-wired species-typical defensive responses to threats that promote survival (Moskowitz, 2004). It is often activated as an aftermath of attachment trauma as the most important trigger of maladaptive activation of the fear-defense systems that may complicate the disorganization of attachment patterns.

There is, in addition, a large complex literature that identifies conflicts in the dynamics of emerging independent and competitive behavior that are often coexisting factors of mental illness. When social interactions or mental events activate the competitive behavior locus, the subject can perceive himself or herself as "destined to victory" or "doomed to defeat," activating either behaviors or emotions connected to the Involuntary Defeat Strategy or Involuntary Dominant Strategy (Johnson, Leedom, and Muhtadie, 2012). In mood or anxiety disorders, physiological and mental consequences of social interaction or inactions occur in both dominants and subordinates but are more extreme in the subordinate. The complex stimulation of adolescent developments likely created strong conflicts in D, (Douglas) who exhibited separate dominant and subordinate entities in his inner world.

While these multiple conflicts in his inner world may be understood from a neuropsychological perspective as emerging because of internally stimulated intense fear and anxiety that generated massive withdrawal into a fragmented inner world, such information is not a guide for therapy. Massive psychic withdrawal, being gone, as described by many authors in catatonia, is the manner a weakened ego protects the individual in the face of total psychological collapse. Moskowitz (2004) hypothesized that the neurological origin of the massive catatonic withdrawal is likely a primitive prey response to fear or extreme stress, analogous to the tonic immobility defense strategy in certain animals. Caught between extreme external threat and internal danger, the vulnerable person withdraws into autistic encapsulation: the closure of direct contact with reality as a partial solution to survival.

While researchers generally focused on the dynamics of attachment, Ogden speculated on a preliminary stage from which attachment emerges. Psychic withdrawal for Ogden (1989), following Bick's ideas, is elaborated as a primary position that they believe exists developmentally prior to the usual paranoid-schizoid and depressive' positions. Referred to by Grotstein (1987) as the "autistic-contiguous" position as a primary "sensory floor" of experience upon which the emerging experience of self becomes elaborated. It may also be a fundamental stage or position responsive prior to the internal benefits and awareness of sensory attachment from the beginning of life. It is a primary stage attuned to the most elemental form of pre-symbolic human experience of safety (touch, closeness, and gaze) and to its absence. Mitrani (1992) prefers the concept of delusion as a concrete event in describing her similar findings in extended therapy with non-neurotic patients who fill emptiness with concrete delusional objects in a manner like D's malignant "NoBody."

One important absence in this original narrative of treatment is an understanding of the original forces compelling such a drastic retreat. This problem is raised by Karyn Todes in her discussion of D's fire setting.

References

Coen, S. J. (2000) Why We Need to Write Openly About Our Clinical Cases. *Journal of the American Psychoanalytic Association* 48:449–470.

Giacolini, T. and Sabatello, U. (2019) Psychoanalysis and Affective Neuroscience. The Motivational/Emotional System of Aggression in Human Relations. *Frontiers in Psychology* 9:2475.

Grotstein, J., Solomon, M. F., and Lang, J. A. (1987) *The Borderline Patient: Emerging Concepts in Diagnosis, Psychodynamics and Treatment.* London: Routledge.

Johnson, S. L., Leedom, L. J., and Muhtadie, L. (2012) The Dominance Behavioral System and Psychopathology: Evidence from Self-Report, Observational, and Biological Studies. *Psychological Bulletin* 138:692–743.

Mitrani, J. L. (1992) On the Survival Function of Autistic Manoeuvres in Adult Patients. *The International Journal of Psychoanalysis* 73:549–559.

Moskowitz, A. (2004) "Scared Stiff": An Evolutionary-Based Fear Response. *Psychological Review* 18:984–1002.

Ogden, T. H. (1989) *The Primitive Edge of Experience.* New York: J. Aronson.

1 Early case of therapy with a catatonic boy

Bennett E. Roth

From Alice in Wonderland: imagination is the only weapon in the war against reality

The imaginative faculty is an essential element in art, music, and science, and somehow, it goes terribly awry in certain mental conditions. Bleuler (1912) described disorders of imaginary life in his pioneer descriptions of schizophrenia disorders as early as 1911 in which there is a complex symptom combining a detachment from reality with a withdrawal into an internal fantasy life.

Rasmussen and Parnas (2018) claimed that psychiatry lacks the conceptual and descriptive resources to grasp the specificity of the imaginative life of patients. In addition, the frequently used term "inner world" is somewhat vague and begs clarification. For example, does the experience of an inner mental life have dimensions? Is it layered or empty? In the following, the inner world of an adolescent boy is reconstructed, and although I was naïve at the time, you may use this data to uncover a new understanding of his illness, its representation, and similar presence in other severe illnesses. I came to understand that his phantasy, imagination, and perception were not only unusual modes of mental events but also, and more importantly, different *strata* or layers of private experience. Briefly, perception is a response to a presence, imagination with private representation, and phantasy with a non-positional appearance of something that is neither present nor represented by the senses. Each mental event may be considered real to him whether it arises from the system unconscious or consciousness and whether constructive or destructive. It is assumed that the boys' imaginative internal world attempted to resolve some internal conflict and was antagonistic to elements of his reality.

History

I was a staff psychologist assigned to a female children's unit and had been there maybe for 13 months. The young girls on my unit were quite disturbed, more so than the boys but that is a different story. Larry and Peter were on an experimental unit for adolescents that were being prepared for discharge.

DOI: 10.4324/9781003427049-2

They both were in a class with me in New School that I enrolled in to meet the requirements for taking the examination to work as a psychologist at a state hospital. Their unit was created after there was a revision of the commitment law for children in New York State. Previously, a child could be committed to a mental hospital and be there for life. The law was changed to require recommitted at the age of 18 as an adult. The administrations searched to find children wrongly committed or somehow remarkably better that would not earn a commitment. That was Larry and Pete's unit. What did I want from them? What was I hoping for? A nonpsychotic adolescent able to relate and talk in therapy as the regular children's unit I was assigned to held no such child.

You may wonder at this point whether I had any training in therapy, and the answer was not at all. I was working in a local clinic in Queens trying to get experience and supervision in psychotherapy. As best I knew, it was getting people to talk to me honestly and emotionally; I got that part right. I was assigned several silent, seemingly numb preadolescent boys with absent fathers. I guess it was relationship therapy of some kind because eventually they began to talk. One boy I took to the local Burger King and he cried that I cared enough to "spend money" on him. Pesky at the hospital finally Larry responded with a name Douglas or D hereafter.

The therapy was to start Monday in the two-story building that housed the experimental adolescent unit, its schoolroom, and wards. I was to go and call out his name in the Rec room filled with State requisitioned tables and chairs with adolescence of every description talking to each other. After the uni-sex wards, it took a moment to get used to. I called out his name loudly looking around the room for a reply of some kind. No visible response. I tried one more time and then a pale thin blond boy stood up with a fixed smile on his face. He did not turn to face me and I walked in front of him and repeated his name. There was no response of recognition. It took a moment to sink in. . . . He was catatonic.[1] We walked to the door leading to the private room I was assigned, and he walked like a toy soldier. Coming to the door, he still walked in place in front of the closed door. I reached around him to open the door and had to move him back a few steps so the door could open. I registered nothing but my mind was racing wondering if Larry and Pete were watching. Watching and laughing at me.

The room was part of an attic as it had a sharply angled slanted roof with a table and two chairs across its wide beam. D stood ramrod tall, and I pointed at the chair and that elicited no response. I debated whether to make him sit down physically and decided that touching him was not a good idea. So I sat and he stood the entire time. When I opened the door 35 minutes later, we were in the same position, and somehow when the door opened, he marched out in the same manner as he marched in. I walked through the rec room back to my office. I said nothing about the incident and acted in my usual manner.

I looked up "catatonia" in the psychiatric books, and whatever I read offered little hope for any form of psychotherapy. No point producing it here. . . . I could not understand how he had been moved to a program that was preparing adolescents for discharge. I went back two days later as planned. Larry watched me enter the rec room and D march "out the door" with me as I held it open. D stood in front of the chair, and I sat down. Took out a pack of gum, opened it, put a piece in my mouth, and offered one to D. No response. I sat back in the chair. Moved his chair toward me and put one leg on it and waited. Time went by slowly, and I soothed myself as I developed a plan that I would stay five weeks, ten sessions, and then leave. I would make Larry curious about what was happening. I would not confide in anyone as to the real nature of the interaction.

I continued to show up for sessions and began to relax and enjoy the time alone in the room with D. I was alone, and he made no demands on me. My mind wandered. I thought of my recent vacation in Mexico as a honeymoon. The interesting people I met in Cuernavaca. Reflected on the interesting people and political discussions at lunch. Still adjusting to living with someone and being married. I was the newest staff member and began thinking again of trying to get a Ph.D. as I had secured the unlikely praise of Dr. Loretta Bender, the child consultant to the hospital. I had also been bumped out of the children's unit despite the wish of the chief psychiatrist that I be put in charge of that small staff of psychologists. I wondered what and where else I could get a job. I was at that hospital over a year and the reception unit was not as busy as the children's unit had been and there was lots of free time. Two weeks passed in this situation and I sat silently: I was relaxed and preoccupied with my own fantasies and thoughts while D sat rigidly in the chair. In the third week we assumed out usual act and I was in my thoughts and I looked at him and he "seemed to roll his tongue out at me leaving it out." Having 4 nephews that I baby-sat for I reflexively stuck my fatter tongue out at him: leaving it out. He then said, "Who told you to do that?"

I said, "Who told you to do that?"
He said, "Nobody told me."
I said, "Nobody told me."
He said, "You speak to nobody?"
I said, "You speak to nobody?"
He said, "Nobody speaks to me."
I said, "No body speaks to me"
He said, "Nobody tells me what to do"
I said, "No body tells me what to do or say"
He laughed and said, "Nobody tells me what to say."

I wasn't sure what had happened. He was silent for more than two years. He stuck his tongue out again and I did too. And the rec alarm sounded that he had to return. He walked his usual walk out the door when opened.

I did not think I could explain what had started him talking. He had an adolescent high-pitched voice and had looked me in the face. I thought it was totally beyond any understanding at that time. I told no one what had happened.

I has no explanation lr9oe for n what had just happened and he had an adolescent high-pitched voice and had looked me in the face. I thought it was totally beyond any understanding at that time. I told no one what had happened.

In the next session, he stuck his tongue out at me again, and we repeated the sequence of words focused on the different meaning of the name "Nobody." In addition, his facial muscles contorted before he spoke as if there were opposing forces in his face to keep his mouth shut. I could not put any meaning together nor did I understand what he was saying beyond its surface meaning. In the third session, he sat down in the chair, and I said "Nobody talks to you" and his fixed smile got wider. I tried a few statements and then came up with, "Where is Nobody?" He said "Gone." And I repeated "Where is nobody gone?" He said "Gone. Nowhere"

In the third session after talking, he sat down in the chair in front of me looking very uncomfortable and stiff. I asked him "How are you?" and he did not respond. I waited and said, "Where is nobody?" And he said, "Gone". I repeated the word gone, and he said "No where." I repeated the words "No where" and he nodded his head once. I had leaned toward him and realized that I was tense and I sat back. His demeanor did not change. We lapsed into silence.

After the session, I searched in the psychoanalytic journals that had accrued in my office as part of the circulating library at the hospital. Looking for any article on treating psychotic patients, there were very few. But I felt encouraged although I was not sure about anything that was happening. He was talking, and I was trying to stay in verbal contact with him.

Next session, he sat stiffly in the chair, and I had moved the chair closer, so we were only 5–6 feet apart. "Where is nobody?" I began. "Gone," was his reply.

"When does he come back?" I asked.
"He comes right back At night."
"No body comes right back at night . . ."
"No body doesn't like you."
"No body knows about me."
"No body knows you talk to me."
I am aware that he said I talk to him not he talks to me "He knows about me talking."
"Nobody wants me to be quiet."
"Nobody doesn't like me."

He laughed (this became a repetitive theme) for some sessions. Essentially that No Body felt my interference. The next three sessions had the same sequences starting with No body.

On the way through the rec room the next week, a man who introduced himself as D's occupational therapist stopped me. He said that D had night terrors and woke up screaming, and he thought I should know about this. I thanked him, shook his hand, and went on to the session. His screaming was described as having been while he was still asleep, and I did not immediately know how to bring this up to D. It was information from outside the sessions.

He had mentioned in a session that "Nobody" appears at night. I could ask if he was frightened of Nobody. There were lots of issues but mostly I was getting enmeshed in his inner world and his language. I was thinking of no body as a thing of some kind. I would soon think of Nobody as directing him as I discovered in his record that after he set his home on fire, he was asked, "Who told you to do that?" And it was reported in his case record that he replied with a smile "Nobody."

At this point, I had no organized plan or sense of the direction of my relationship with D. Larry and Peter retreated in my mind. I was starting to battle confusion after his sessions about his negative language. My verbal exchanges with D affected my use of language after the sessions. As we continued, this became more of a problem. Frank V. noticed my pre-occupation and asked about its source. I replied that it was from D's therapy sessions. He volunteered to listen to me talk it out and later suggested that I tape sessions. I began taping sessions and listening to them with Frank making a list of his words and their meanings as they emerged in the sessions. I soon had 20–25 words that D and I used; most of them were negative and some that had two opposite meaning.

The following is a condensation of the dynamics of treatment. D said to me, "Can you do this?" And he opened his mouth and rolled his tongue like a lizard tasting the air. I stuck my tongue out and tried to move it and made gross movements. D laughed silently at me. I would see that tongue often tasting the air. D continued this behavior, and it was never interpreted, as I had no idea other than it was somehow protective. I knew nothing of the neurological underpinning of the ability. Later it would occur with great intensity in a dramatic episode.

"Where is No body" I began
"He is gone"
"Where is No body?"
"He is gone"
"Where is gone?"
"I am gone."
"You are Gone"
"You are Gone?" I repeat.

At this time, I realized that his last name had the same sound as Gone and that this had more than one meaning. It was a homophone. And so I had repeated the phrase.

"You are gone"
He replied, "I am gone now."
"You are gone now," I repeated without knowing what it meant to him, thinking that gone now was different from gone.
"I was blind," he continued.
I was surprised by the term and hesitated.

"Blind?"
"I was blind."
"Blind" "You can't see?"
"I was blind. I won't be right back."
I figured out right back was here present but here with me? Or just here. Did gone now mean he was himself? I was confused.

Another vignette "Where were you?" I asked.
"I was gone".
"You were gone?"
"I was no where."
(I thought I caught on) where is nowhere?
"Not here. I am not here. I am nowhere."
"No where" "No where, not here is where you are."
"I won't be right back."
"Ok; No where, not here, right back. Blind."

I was invited by his Occupational therapist to see a clay figure D made from a drawing. The drawing was quite talented and explicit. It had a large-beaked bird's head like an eagle on a huge bear like frame, with alligator feet and large lobster claws for hands. I was silent and the OT was instructing D to take a hammer and attack the clay figure they had made together. I tried to stop him by waving my hands as I had agreed to not speak. The OT brushed me off insisting that it was therapeutic. D took a hammer and destroyed the clay figure smiling and sticking his tongue out. I left the OT room anxious for him. D missed the next two sessions and was catatonic again. He had gone to sleep, woke up screaming and became rigid again. On the third session after the event, he was walked to the session by an orderly in his familiar gate. He didn't talk till the next session.

I waited for him to talk, and he was silent, and I said, "No body came"
He replied, "He was a message."
"He was a message?"
"He was a message."
"What message?"
"No body will kill you?"
"No body wants to kill me? Or kill you?"
"No body will kill you. I won't be right back"
"I am not afraid of NO body" (verbal exaggeration)
"No body will kill you"
"I am not afraid of No body"
"Be afraid"
(Long pause)

"Where are you no body? Don't hide from me. Come on out. Show yourself don't be no where."

I stand up and I do an imitation of Burt Lahr as the Cowardly Lion.

Oh Yea come on out and I will fight you. I aint afraid of you. I aint afraid of no body. No body come on and fight me. Come on out. Don't hide you coward. I will fight you with one hand behind my back (I am standing now and assume a boxer's stance) Come on out you nobody. You are afraid nobody. Show yourself. Don't hide; I will fight you with two hands behind my back.

Shuffling into boxer stance. "You're the one afraid," and then I do an Ali shuffle. "Come on out you mangy coward and fight me. Sting like a bee, float like a butterfly. I am the greatest."

D looks unafraid, smiles, and says, "No body will get you."

I did not know what to anticipate in the next session, I told Dr. V. I had a break through understanding that "No body" meant having no body and only a voice. No physical body. A voice talked to him without a body. I suspect it gave him orders. I told him about the threat but now did not understand who was really making the threat. D or no body. "Be right back" didn't mean he would be there; sometimes it meant the opposite that he was disappeared. Gone was a place in his mind but also was close in sound to his name. No where was where "No body went" when he could not hear him.

I come to the session, and when he sees me, D was smiling, and I say, "Here I am"; and he replies, "You are; Ben equally strong the way he is." He renamed me.
"No body is afraid of me." I tell him.
He replies, "You can't see" No body. He only speaks to me, "This I hear as confirmation that "No body" is just a voice he hears. Nobody is just a voice and sometimes the voice is the source of the message." "Where is No body?" I ask.
"Not here" is his reply.
"Where is not here" I ask. I think "Not here" and "Nowhere" are different places
"Not here or No where" I ask.
"He is not here?" I ask. And I suddenly realized that "Not Here" is a place in his mind. It had double meaning. He was in "not here" and he was not present. Within the next 2 weeks I discovered a host of places and another voice: a very large parakeet that spoke without its beak moving. Not present, no where, "not here" were places that no body was when he wasn't

talking to D. He often replied to the question; Where were you? No where or no place, not here. . . . [T]hese were his hiding places in his mind where the creature or creatures that attacked him could not get to him. I did not know if he or no body could hide there. He might reply, "I am not here" to a question and then asked where he was. He answered, "Not here." If he said I am not here sometimes he was invisible. If he said I am blind he meant, "You can't see me." Was no body a protector or an attacker? I did not know. "Not here" I understood as if he was inside a box and the outside was where reality started. When he was inside the layered box what was he? I wondered if when he said he was blind he thought that I could not see him because he was nowhere. Agent and agency were also confused as was active and passive. I made up a chart of places and names and it numbered more than 25. For another example "When he used" Be right back" he was obscuring the fact that elements (whatever it was) were disintegrated. If I asked "back yet?" in some form he might only smile. What was the role of promises? There was no past tense everything was in the present.

I suffered a strange form of confusion after sessions as I had to use D's vocabulary to communicate and continued to play the tapes for Dr. V. Also, Dr. V was very clear in that he did not intrude in what was taking place in the therapy or in the dialogue but gently questioned me as to what I thought and felt in the sessions. In one session, I said: "I think I am being misled by 'no body.' I think it's something devious and he is hiding from me by inventing other names." D also told me that he had "torn the head off his mother's parakeet" because he thought the birds' noise was telling his mother what he had done in the bathroom. Initially, I thought he was masturbating but then I was unsure. Was he reading something? I confronted D and told him that Nobody was hiding and inventing names to fool me. He smiled.

Meanwhile, D started attending school although he did not speak while there. He sat with other people at lunch and seemed awkward. I was informed of these two changes later by the chief psychiatrist.

I was asked by the same OT man to take D outside the ward. He had not been outside the hospital for two years. He was given some money, and I was to take him to the canteen to buy some food. I agreed and we walked outside the ward. D was obviously nervous and shaking and I asked if he wanted to hold me arm. He did not reply but did. We eventually walked to the canteen and he again could not speak. I asked him what he wanted and he just looked at me. I said soda, candy, and chips, and he did not respond. I said them again and he nodded at soda. I took the bottle and said, "You have to pay." It took three times asking for him to pay. I took the top off the soda and he took a long drink and held the bottle all the way back in two hands.

Our third trip to the canteen was dramatic. As we turned the corner of the building, there was a dead sea gull on the ground. The hospital was on the shore of the South Bay. D stopped and stared at it. As we turned the next corner he started to shake physically and look back. He half turned as if to go back and I verbalized, "You have to go back." He turned and walked back stiffly and stopped about 4 feet from the bird and stared at it. He then began to roll his tongue at it and make up and down gestures with his hands and dance around the bird. I moved to continually face him bisecting the space and decided to copy his gestures as best I could while thinking that "I did not want to leave him alone." We were both arm waving and moving in a circle around the bird on the ground when he opened his fly and peed on the bird. So I did the same. Eventually, he stopped moving, and we went to the canteen and he held my arm and ordered by himself. He had stopped shaking. I took a different route to his ward to avoid the dead bird.

Upon my return to my office Dr. V was waiting for me and smiling said, "What did you do?" "Why"? I responded and he said. "The chief psychiatrist called and said you had to be fired." "Damm," I said and told V about the event. V said "He said he saw you out his window." V suggested that we take the tape recorder and tapes and go to the doctors' office and we played the tapes for him. V went to talk to him alone. What was in my favor was that V was on my side and D was recovering. After V came out we both went in and I explained about the night terrors and the attacking bird. That chief psychiatrist was looking at me as oddly but I held my ground, and he relented mostly because of D's recovery; however, every time I came to the ward, I had to check in with him and to promise to not do such a thing again. In the meantime, the Assistant Director of the Hospital was informed of the incident and suggested to V that I treat his niece who was in a major depressive episode. V and I walked back to the psych unit, and he was laughing saying. "Thank God we have the tapes of the nightmare bird. Did you see his face how he looked at you?" V never questioned anything that I did. And shortly after this event he suggested that I have lunch with him and the man who I had replaced who was in a Ph.D. program at NYU. V suggested that he recommend me to the chairperson and that was a step toward my leaving. In addition, after four sessions the young girl with a major depression began to groom and clean herself although I later thought it was a romantic cure. Throughout her sessions, I thought and did not say out loud "Get out of my office you stink." When I left, the assistant director did not let me resign my position and gave me a year's leave of absence. D was discharged without any effort to consult me. I went to the unit to watch him leave and his mother anxiously looked like a bird to me as she moved around him.

The tapes of D's sessions and my tape recorder were stolen from my first office although hidden in a compartment under the Swedish day bed couch I was using. After I started analytic training while reading Freud's cases, I thought that he never met the patients in their craziness but remained outside of their experience. His explanations and interpretations seemed outside their box not inside. I caused a major stir among the faculty and I was surprised by their case presentations. Training pushed me outside of the patient's world to making interpretations that never seemed to have any effect. I did however present some of that clinical experience with D to Dr. Bion in a consultation and he responded to the nightmare animal wondering what he had seen that his eyes were attacked. I was still more interested in the monsters parts. Years later, I thought of Bion's remark as focused on the punishment of Oedipus at Clonus.

I will attempt to establish a theoretical foundation for what transpired in D's aborted therapy by employing the concept of *pathological organization*, a term that has been used by various psychoanalytic authors. I hope to gain a better understanding of D's personality disturbances and the dynamics of his partial recovery (Hinshelwood, 1991). Briefly, imaginative experience is characterized by unreality, ipseity (first-person perspective "mineness" of experience), and interiority. His experience took place in a different dimension of social reality.

It is important not to confuse the notion of an external mage with an object of "inner perception" or attention. This mistake is coined as an "illusion of immanence." Contrary to a perceived object illusory objects are private. My idea of the unconscious, as Meltzer describes, is emotional rather than geometric and composed of internal objects and infantile fragments of the self. My analytic theory is (among others) based on Klein's early observation that...

"if persecutory fears are very strong, and for this reason . . . the infant cannot work through the later developmental progressions. From this theory the working through of the negative position is in turn impeded. Think separation fears. This failure may lead to a regressive reinforcing of persecutory fears and strengthen the fixation points for severe psychoses."

(1952, p. 294)

(An adult male patient had persisting night terrors of a giant woman outside his house waiting for him and slept with the TV and lights on.) O'Shaughnessy's (1981) concept of the *defensive organization* emphasizes this pathological fixation among children, who, because of a "weak ego" and the experience of extreme persecution anxieties, fail to develop a stable identity or have malignant attachment issues. Their ego-development stagnates in the defensive mechanisms typical of a negative paranoid-schizoid position. Such stagnation leads either to an immature psychic equilibrium or to an extremely narcissistic personality structure organized around omnipotent defensive mechanisms. Based on Bion's (1957) differentiation of psychotic and nonpsychotic parts of the personality and the splitting that goes along with this, Meltzer (1968) and Money-Kyrle (1969) metaphorically described an internal quarrel between the healthy and sick parts of the self. A quarrel between D and Nobody and Ben-equally-strong. This quarrel seemed to occur in the second phase as I represented an aspect of attention to reality as Ben Equally strong. Often this discovered internal element could also be projected into the outer world of the environment (Segal, 1956) rather than subjected to a splitting of bad and good parts. Steiner (1989, 1993), on the other hand, writes that pathological organizations are mainly characterized by a kind of "emotional geography or "liaison of fragments' under the dominance of an omnipotent narcissistic component which itself is the result of failed splitting. Lawrence (2000) relying on Bion's description of psychosis in general as the process whereby humans defend themselves from understanding the meaning and significance of reality, because they regard such knowing as painful. To do this, they use aspects of their mental functioning to destroy, in various degrees, the very process of thinking that would allow them to be in touch with reality.

In D, this did not occur totally but led to a remarkable inability to use language to communicate confusion, distress, or fear until our engagement.

The language and logic in D's interaction and communication that usually emerges with consensual meaning was turned upside down and infused with multiple meanings. Words often varied in their meaning and in some cases were turned into imaginary internal locations and negative dynamics that revealed hidden malignant forces or hiding places. Does this presentation support a notion of splitting and reversal of direction in severe illness? I think, it does. Although I was naïve, is the unusual kind of "negative" force theoretically assumed to be present in psychosis revealed in D? Is the negative omnipotent threatening split off internal aspect revealed by D's "No-body" as the malignant imaginary totalitarian presence in his mind. The bidirectionality of this force as a protector from reality and internal threat was also revealed in his process?

Three last ideas. The classical concepts of holding, containing, and mirroring are relatively broad in their usage resulting in varied interpretations that omit the use and acceptance and openness toward the use of the client's language. The use of the D's language was essential to D's internalization of naming the comic me that requires understanding as a mock battle with an imaginary internal foe. That I survived his imaginary attack must also be significant. Of some importance was the role my honest ignorance played in his treatment.

Note

1 Catatonia is a mental state of apparent unresponsiveness to external stimuli and apparent inability to move normally in a person who is apparently awake. There are three types: (1) catatonia associated with another mental disorder (catatonia specifier), (2) catatonic disorder due to another medical condition, and (3) unspecified catatonia. Once thought to be related to schizophrenia it is now thought to be related to a range of affective disorders.

References

Bion, W. R. (1957) Differentiation of the Psychotic from Non-Psychotic Personalities. *The International Journal of Psychoanalysis* 38:266–275.

Bleuler, E. (1912) The Theory of Schizophrenic Negativism. *The Journal of Nervous and Mental Disease* 39(1):50–57.

Hinshelwood, R. D. (1991) Psychodynamic Formulation in Assessment for Psychotherapy. *British Journal of Psychotherapy* 8:166–174.

Klein, M. (1952) Some Theoretical Conclusions regarding the Emotional Life of the Infant. In: *The Writings of Melanie Klein, Volume 8: Envy and Gratitude and Other Works*. London: Hogarth Press, pp. 61–94.

Lawrence, W. G. (2000) Thinking Refracted. In W. G. Lawrence (ed.) *Tongued with Fire. Groups in Experience*. London: Karnac, pp. 1–30.

Meltzer, D. (1968) Terror, Persecution, Dread: A Dissection of Paranoid Anxieties. *The International Journal of Psychoanalysis* 49(2–3):396–401.

Money-Kyrle, R. (1969) *Collected Papers of Roger Money-Kyrle*. R. Harris Educational Trust Library Series # 7. Karnac Books, London.

O'Shaughnessy, E. (1981) A Clinical Study of a Defensive Organization. *International Journal of Psychoanalysis* 62:359–428. Republished in Spillus E. *Melanie Klein Today*, Vol. 2. Routledge (1988).

Rasmussen, A. R., and Parnas, J. (2018) Anomalies of Imagination and Disordered Self in Schizophrenia Spectrum Disorder. Psychopathology. 48:317–323.

Segal, H. (1956) Depression in the Schizophrenic. *International Journal of Psychoanalysis* 37:339–343.

Steiner, J. (1987) The Interplay between Pathological Organisations and the Paranoid-Schizoid and Depressive Positions. *International Journal of Psychoanalysis* 58:69–80. Reprinted in Spillius, E. (1988) *Melanie Klein Today*. Taylor & Frances/Routledge.

Steiner, J. (1993) *Psychic Retreats: Pathological Organization in Psychotic, Neurotic and Borderline Patients*. Routledge. London.

2 Interview with the therapist

Bennett E. Roth

This case report was the unexpected product of a series of events that ordinarily would not lead to any hope or expectancy of a book becoming its end product. A reconstruction of an early encounter with a catatonic boy was originally intended for a psychiatry seminar. It was an unusual and a formative event in my becoming a psychoanalyst and a psychotherapist. The reproduction of this aborted encounter became a vehicle to engage with other professionals interested in working with deeply compromised individuals.

A basic sense of D emerges in the original presentation of his self or adolescent identity being under psychic attack. While I could not fathom the source of the attack, I did not seek to add to his burden. As P. Williams recognized assisting the severely troubled person . . . "while avoiding violation of that person's vulnerable self (identity) is a highly complex undertaking because basic trust is missing" (2022, p. 9): and I must append that threat is experienced as inescapable. Nothing that I did with D conforms with any conventional theories, and my behavior and my thinking appear to touch among different theories of which I was unaware.

Interview with the therapist

The questions in my interview that follow are influenced by a variety of psychoanalytic sources. In particular, I am influenced by a chapter in "War Memories" (1997), where Bion, as a psychoanalyst, constructed a dialogue with Bion as a soldier in WWI. In the following, I am conferring with my earlier self, revealing that earlier version of myself who engaged this boy. When I constructed this case study, I relied on trying to capture the essence of the person I was then without being consciously influenced by further experience and learning. The reconstruction of the case was facilitated by my memories of its uniqueness.

DOI: 10.4324/9781003427049-3

Interview

When do you think therapy began with D?

Our interactive verbal relationship begins with D challenging me by asking, in response to sticking my tongue at him after he did that to me by asking "Who told you to do that?" Something must have happened before that gesture for him to risk speaking to me. My verbal reply in kind was, "Who told you?" His sudden speaking interrupted our familiar silence and broke into my reverie. His tone of adolescent bravado did not match his physical appearance setting up a constant contradiction in the sessions between his physical appearance and internal threats. His tongue came out many times. From that moment on, I was engaged in trying to communicate with him and then in deciphering the meaning of his vocabulary. I was almost immediately aware that we did not share a common reference for his "nobody" in the opening sentences. I was not initially aware of the complexity of D's language and often was confused in sessions when trying to communicate to him and establish that I was independent from him. Presciently aware, I sensed that the threat of "Nobody" for D was psychically real as he made his fear known to me. The actual nature of the threat remained unrevealed. The report from the occupational therapist of night terrors confirmed the presence of an internal threat but he did not mention them other than his eyes being attacked. Being "recognized" by Nobody as being in competition for D was also a surprise as he was attributing motive to what I thought was his mental image. Nobody was a voice without a body. I had no experience with an internal voice giving orders. It was all new to me.

What did you make of his tongue behavior?

Over time, I had different ideas of his tongue coming out. Initially I wasn't initially sure he rolled his tongue out or I imagined it. In the early sessions he did it frequently and I assumed it was "tasting the environment to see if it was safe." When he stuck out his tongue continuously at the dead bird, I thought it was protective magic and in place of speaking. After the dead bird incident, it stopped happening.

Did you inquire about its absence?

I asked very few questions in general despite his speech being filled with constantly changing terms in his negative language. His inner world of named places was always changing, and he was adapting to leaving the ward. I tried to make short clear statements.

Did you think anything of the dynamics of his becoming psychotic?

Not really. I knew nothing about his past except for reading the information in his medical record. He only made reference to the parakeet he killed, by tearing its head off, he believed for revealing something the bird said to his mother. That was clearly paranoid violence and indicated the possible presence of "secrets." I thought he had a secret world in his mind. He never admitted what he thought the parakeet said and I never asked. In addition, I was never sure he knew what was true or real or not.

With disturbed patients, there are usually crises that occur in treatment. What were your crises?

The first crises were the destruction of the clay figure in the OT. I suddenly realized that Nobody would retaliate in some manner for the attack on the figure. It still seems odd to refer to "no body" as an entity. I experienced a sudden apprehension in the OT that something was going to happen to D if the clay figure was of "Nobody" and was attacked. I promised to be silent and I did not want to intrude, as it seemed that OT was in a place he felt able to play and be safe without speaking. The clay creature he made fascinated me. I read a paper on splitting and tried to understand how the animal elements were formed together as a whole image. At first, familiar with totem poles, I thought it combined elements of the parts of the different animals that signified parts of him. It made no sense to me except that it was dangerous. The OT thought it was a nightmare figure and thought it could be removed or damaged by symbolically destroying it. After the event, D became catatonic for a short time.

Another crises began with D telling me to be afraid of "Nobody" meaning, I thought, that he too was afraid. I had begun to recognize the centrality of "Nobody" in his internal world and often though of the verbal game "who's there? Nobody but us chickens." I read about splitting as a defense but did not recognize that his was a punitive fragment of D. "Nobody" never spoke directly to me. D did not speak in another voice. I became spontaneous in response to the "threat" conveyed by D in a comic theatrical response perhaps sensitive to what happened in the OT.

My comic turn as the *Cowardly Lion* from the Wizard of Oz had multiple meanings not the least was that D smiled at my theatrics. I was pleased by a frightened boy's smile. I had done a similar imitating of the actor Burt Lahr in voice and movements with my young nephews, and they laughed too. The double meanings of the character were clear to me that I was both a threat and no threat and I was part Theater. Calling out "Nobody" to appear and not hide was a challenging way of demonstrating that he wasn't on "the outside" and in reality and in particular real to me. It was a first grounding of a distinction of inside and outside for D and once again he smiled as I did a poor demonstration of M Ali. I was playing the role that I was the champ, unafraid, and I was the equal of "Nobody." Perhaps looking back on the event it might seem absurd to some observers but humor and absurdity are often neglected in recovery. D's face was more child-like when he smiled. I think the realization that "No Body" did not hurt me was the turning point of his getting better. Maybe, that I may be able to protect him.

The accidental encounter with the dead sea gull led to a crises for D. Looking back at that event now I recognize and am surprised at how potentially dangerous that situation was. If he became psychotic, we were on the path to the canteen with no help immediately available if that happened. I would need to bring him back to the ward by myself. I was until now unaware of this. It was never brought to my attention by other staff. What I recall was responding to him as he became anxious and preoccupied looking back at the site with the dead bird. He was starting to physically tremble, and I asked in a directive way if he wanted to go back. I assumed that he needed to see that the body of the bird was still there and to see it again. I was highly alert to him as he approached the bird body and stood opposite him. I began to copy his behavior without any decision to do so. I kept the same distance between us as he circled the carcass to not intrude in his space and felt no shame in joining him urinating on the carcass. He calmed down after a few turns and urinating. He didn't look at me when we were able to return to the ward and took my arm. On the way to my office I was still highly alert and trying to understand what happened. I often had transition problems after a session. I was trying to process what happened and transition to "normal" language while recovering emotionally from sessions.

Did you know of "mirroring": as a technique?

No I found that later.

Is being so alert important to you? You keep mentioning it.

Yes, I was an athlete into my twenties and when I was athletic, I was very focused and alert to the situations in a ballgame. I learned to take everything and everyone in and respond to it without conscious thought. If you think in a game it is often too late to act. Nothing else existed in that room but D and me, in particular after the threat and also with the dead bird. I did not consciously choose to revive my imitation of Burt Lahr. It happened. As I think of it now I was creating an illusion, creating a pretend person to challenge his dangerous pretend person. Theater and movies are an illusion without a real threat.

You were meeting his illusion with your constructed illusion.

My illusions were comic and strong . . . his were dangerous.

Were you concerned about being fired from your position?

Initially, I was surprised being told that someone viewed the dance I did with D. Frank V. being calm and treating the matter with a smile and without much emotion was my guide. I was not confident in the Medical Doctors at the hospital. Most of them had little experience and were in their residency. None of them, to my knowledge, were interested in psychotherapy of any kind. I had very little contact with the medical director of that adolescent unit other than noticing that he dressed well. He was really upset by what he witnessed me doing out of the ward. Dr. V cautioned me to remain quiet and only answer questions. I don't think I would be able to explain what I did other than to admit that I did not want him to be alone and in danger. That he was not catatonic after returning to the ward was the persuasive element in his decision.

It appears that you were in a different mental state when you were with D.

It was a new experience and an unusual one for me. It was unchartered territory. Even to say that is odd or incorrect as I had so little experience being a therapist. I tried to be open to him and receive information. Often I was puzzled by what had occurred in my conversations with D. as we were in his inner world. I initially did not know that "no body" was an entity in his mind. And then that he experienced no body as being able to hide or attack him. I did not know what No body's power was over him? I also encountered other terms *of No where, Not here, no place* that were treated as places by him, that I assumed were "places" to him. I tried to imagine his mind as if a physical space in which there was movement or traffic. He could see inside or sense internal entities as if in a waking dream. I thought that is what psychosis was: a waking dream. Then, it was as if some normalizing energy appeared in him. I was also surprised that he started to socialize. I think I did not think he would be related and discharged. It was all new to me. The hardest part of his therapy for me was using his negative language. I had to speak slowly always translating into his vocabulary until I thought he was fooling me.

You confronted him about fooling you.

Yes, I was trying to understand him and it felt like he was leading me into places with negative names that would then disappear or not be there a second time. I tried to follow his words from session to session and had the sudden thought that he was tricking me. I didn't think there was any motive other than to mislead me. So I confronted him and he smiled when I told him that I thought it was "No body" fooling me and to tell me the most important names. We continued with those names.

Do you consider yourself a creative therapist?

For creative therapists,[1] every case is a new experience. Not as Bion puts it as a sense of the therapist being "without memory or desire," although that maybe what he meant. I do not know what I will encounter and what I will be called on to understand and respond to when engaged with someone seeking psychic change. I think I am unafraid when doing this work. I was afraid only once that I remember and was not afraid with D. Because I had no training in psychotherapy I relied on my prior experience of trying to establish trust with the person and understanding their communication.

How did you understand D from a psychological perspective?

I originally had a very few separate ideas about him once he started to talk. He seemed at one time to be intelligent and then something happened and he, as an entity, disappeared. I believe he reached out to me because of my sticking my tongue out and asked a question that focused my full attention to him. His language was unique and deceptive and emerged as if a game or puzzle. I was always uncertain I understood what he said. The negativity in his language was constant and I realized how neutral language was in comparison to his speech. Using his language was confusing to me, it was as if constantly saying no, not or describing a photonegative. I knew that when he said I am "Gone;" it held more than one meaning but it puzzled me. Where was gone? Where was he?

You trusted yourself in the room with him.

I had a pretty strong sense of self, unfinished, as it was and struggled with understanding his vocabulary. His language was also fluid and as if he was talking from a frame of reference we did not share and I could not imagine what he observed. His vision appeared too often to be internal, looking inside of "something" or sensing it and speaking of it as if real to both of us. I was a good diagnostician and was an independent learner and often it felt that while I was with him in the room I was alone. I was in a room with him and only I was trying to understand what was happening. Trusting him was difficult. Many analysts recognize:

> The sense of the unity of the self or of identity that is over and above the classical analytic topographies can be fractured from within or by being unprotected when vulnerable or in development. When that happens self-experience is dislocated, fragmented or split off. Do you agree with that statement?

My experience with D confirms this dynamic of fracture. However, there was more to this than acknowledged by this quote as internal violence appeared among his fractured elements. Whatever was his fracturing process kept attacking other parts of the self. There were at least three other forces against some elements of self. Nobody, the clay creature represented in OT, and the parakeet. There were also night terrors and the fear of the dead bird that played out in his panic. These named internal entities could be obscured, hidden by him but how do you actively hide an idea or a mental image and by what agent or agency? Understanding is needed to decipher the source and dynamics of this negative energy and its targets.

On to D., I never knew how D became withdrawn, his developmental history or his family. I was uninterested in any developmental explanation as I viewed it as unhelpful and unknowable given his mental state. I believed that history was beyond my and his reach. Later I thought, causal explanations in psychoanalysis were speculative usually dependent on the therapist's theoretical orientation. I realized when someone inquired about his relationship with his parents at a presentation, hinting I thought, at possible Oedipal conflicts, that he only mentioned his mother once and never directly referred to his father. I was unaware of that absence until asked, as I was focused on D's immediate situation. I focused on understanding his communication, the meaning of his language and his effort to communicate to me. His fractured inner world became my focus as he revealed it and as I became a figure in his inner experience. At least, I was given a unique name. There were, in addition, at least three demonic elements in his mind that were animated and visualized by him that sought harm.

How did you respond to his being discharged?

I was concerned that he was being returned to the environment that contributed to his illness. I had no power to intervene. I don't think we had a real good-bye, as I wasn't at the graduation held for the unit. It really did feel like the end of something important and it was the first time I was so deeply engaged.

Having such a therapeutic experience must impact you personally and your work.

At first, I was not aware of any impact and there was a mixture of relief and sadness. I was not aware of the degree of mental effort required to talk with him until it stopped. Then, I was tired. At the same time I was aware of the time of our sessions and missed them. I would look at my watch just when it was time to walk to his unit. I continued to read difficult cases and then my life changed. In the Ph.D. program, I was aware that other professionals maintained distance from really disturbed patients. I did not engage in any therapy for the few years I was in graduate school. In analytic training it seemed that there was a distance from the patient and that the patients' pathology was explained at some distance in the patient's past. I seemed more comfortable working in close with what was expressed in the room. I generally assumed that when the patient referred to someone outside of the room there were projections that distorted what the patient was describing.

In addition, I learned to be comfortably fully mentally present in the treatment room as I was with D. While often presenting some transition problems, such alertness allowed me to be aware of the impact of the patient on me. I also needed a time to "digest" the impact of sessions as I had with D. I was helped later by the seminars I attended with Bion as he did not seek to "move away" from patients but somehow stayed in psychic contact with them. I remember a dream I presented to Bion of a man planning to visit his childhood home in Europe. As he approaches his home in a car, he discovers that a bomb destroyed it. I assumed, from the manifest material, that this happened as he walked among the debris in the cavity and then found and picked up burned toys where his room had been. Bion suggested to me that the man was referring to a memory of a psychotic break and the burned toys were his part objects. I came to understand the meaning of such an early dream indicated the likelihood of a fearful apprehension of treatment leading to a psychotic episode with a traumatic memory.

Is there anything you expected that I did not ask?

I am often asked what started him talking? I don't know the answer to that question. I often wonder at D's getting better or that he was no longer catatonic and whether some latent integrating energy was present despite his problems. That energy was waiting for an opportunity to be expressed.

Note

1 I have been called a creative therapist.

References

Bion, W. R. (2015) Wilfred R. Bion: War Memoirs, 1917–1919. edited by Francesca Bion. Karnac Books. London
Paul Williams (1922) The Authority of Tenderness: Dignity and the True Self in Psychoanalysis. Routledge. London

3 Witnessing the patient with psychosis

Eric R. Marcus

This chapter will explore the phenomena of witnessing and its use in the early psychotherapeutic work with the psychotic patient. When first working with a psychotic patient, there may be no therapeutic alliance. This is because the patient's experience of their psychosis is in reality, and their suffering is caused by reality, for which psychological help would be useless. Dr. Roth understood this with his patient and chose to be there with him, meeting regularly in silence. I will call a certain type of being with someone, focused on them, the opportunity for witnessing.

The term witnessing refers to both an inner experience and an interpersonal relationship: the experience of bearing witness, the experience of being witnessed; the experience of a witnessing relationship. This special relationship and its associated experiences and effects have special utility and meaning in the care of the psychotic patient.

The dictionary defines the act of witnessing as: (1) attesting; to a fact; to testify; to attest, (2) a person who saw; firsthand account; (3) a person called upon to observe for testimony as to fact, (4) serving as evidence; and (5) to act as proof thereof (Merriam-Webster's dictionary).

In human events, the witness attests not just to the facts of events but the emotional reaction; the felt experience and therefore the meaning and significance of the event. The meaning experience lived by the patient and observed by the caregiver. That relationship describes the self-experience in the witness and in the witnessed. This is done through our experience of their experience of meaning. In working with psychotic patients, we try to keep the experience of meaning separate from the experience of reality.

Validate means to affirm meaning; to affirm as significant. To give a fact emotional significance is to affirm that its meaning is also a fact. It is important, noteworthy, valid, and significant. Significant means special in its value. The witness proclaims the special meaning for the patient through the understanding of the specific meaning it has to the patient as experienced by the observing and feeling witness.

DOI: 10.4324/9781003427049-4

The problem with psychotic experience is that meaning has become reality. The witness has the tricky problem of affirming the emotional meaning without affirming the reality of the emotional meaning. The witness does that by affirming the emotional meaning in the shared ordinary reality of the nonpsychotic part of the patient.

Witnessing may raise the significance of meaning to the level of sanctity. Sanctification means to consecrate and to make inviolable. The witness helps to sanctify. Sanctification can be used to effect an inner change of valuation and meaning which causes a transformation of self-experience based on a consolidation of a change in the significance of the feeling and of its meaning. The witness catalyzes a change in the meaning of an event and therefore in self-experience and therefore in the self. The witness helps catalyze a transformational experience of the self. This can bring increased observing ego to the patient. It happens because the witness can sanctify the emotional meaning without condensing it with physical reality. This can help the psychotic patient stop struggling with reality and start to understand the meaning of reality.

Sanctification takes place first in the witness. The witness affirms that the experience has important meaning. This helps the patient feel it. A witness creates a sanctuary – a place for sanctification. We do this in the physical setting of quiet and privacy. We do it in ourselves as witnesses. We do it with the patient in the attentive listening that we do, in the invitation for the patient to join us, and in the relationship that is the result.

A sanctum sanctorum in the witness is a quiet and accessible emotional space. This must be a place of privacy, respect, dignity, and honor. This place we create and maintain as witnesses and caregivers for them. Witnessing is our commitment and ability to build in ourselves an emotional safe place where meaning can be recognized by us in order to help it occur for the patient and catalyze a change in themselves. This place we create and maintain is our ability to take in their self-representation of themselves as our object representation of them influenced by but uncontaminated by our self-representation of ourselves. This is the mental capacity of empathic witnessing. This is what we wish to enact in the relationship to them. This is what we wish for them to elicit and develop in them to use for themselves.

But what happens when the illness is in the mind, and especially when the illness captures an area of the mind's reality experience? Emotional reactions can capture reality experience in illnesses of the body, but in the nonpsychotic patient, reality testing is still intact. It is expected that clarifying the boundary between reality and the emotional reaction that is contaminating the reality experience will result in a detoxification of reality experience and therefore of fear. This is what is called interpreting the transference to the illness.

But what happens in psychosis when the reality testing capacity is blocked by the illness? In psychosis, an area of emotional experience has captured an area of reality experience (Marcus, 2017). The result is a delusion if the psychotic condensation is in the cognitive system or a hallucination if it is in the sensory system. Then, the witnessing job is harder. Then, the witness must be witnessing the suffering of that psychotic contamination without the ability to detoxify reality experience. It can seem futile. This futility can cause the witness to withdraw. It takes a special capacity and much therapeutic experience to maintain optimism for the long view (Schafer, 1959).

It also takes the understanding that witnessing of suffering is a step toward helping the patient understand that they are suffering, which is a step toward understanding what is causing their suffering. In the case of psychotic illness, one of the major causes of their suffering is the psychosis itself.

A psychotic patient needs a witnessing experience because part of their reality experience is trapped in the psychosis, and it captures their self-experience. Psychosis calls for a psychological response by the self but that self-response is in danger of becoming captured by the psychotic condensation with reality. Changes in the self are needed to fight the psychotic illness. This may be more obvious at first to the observer. What is needed is an attestation witnessing of the psychotic illness, by way of witnessing the suffering it causes. We try to help isolate the psychosis from the self-first by witnessing the suffering of the self caused by the psychotic illness. We empathize with their suffering, with the nonpsychotic suffering. We must keep separate the meaning to the self from the meaning in psychosis and this will help us keep separate psychotic reality experience in their psychotic condensation from ordinary reality experience in themselves and in us, even when it is still impossible to separate the psychotic condensation itself into ordinary reality experience and ordinary emotional experience.

The Winnicottian "good enough mother" (Winnicott, 1971a) takes in the emotional experience of the baby, "metabolizes" that experience, which means modulating it and linking it to context, and gives it back in digestible form within the context of her responsive relationship to her baby. The mother places the emotional experience in a relationship context of making reality all right, a positive not a negative, a context not a subject. Her behavior reinforces the reality experience emotional experience boundary. Changing the wet diaper. Providing a feeding.

Bion's similar concept was of the container (Bion, 1970), and by this, he meant a container of affect. The container modulates affect intensity, distills affect meaning, places its significance in context of relationships and physical surround, and gives it back together with its links. With the psychotic patient, the witness must in addition be a container of reality.

Winnicott also described the transitional object (Winnicott, 1971). For Winnicott, the transitional object was the baby's "first not me" object. The transitional object was an object in reality that was neither the baby nor the mother. The object could be a blanket, a toy, or the baby's thumb. The crucial issue was that the baby experienced it as a possession under the baby's control, not the mother's. Winnicott's description of the transitional object is a symbolic representation of the mother. But it is also a plaything, an interactional; for the imagination, for fantasy play.

Winnicott described the mental experience of such a plaything as midway between fantasy experience and reality experience. This plaything was therefore transitional between emotional experience and reality experience. This is what he meant by transitional space; a space in the mind for this transitional process to occur. The mother must never question whether the transitional object was found or invented. It is of course both, but the found aspect must never ruin the invented aspect. In this way, the mother is witness to the capacity for transitional experience. Something can be both found and invented, real and imaginary. This is what the witness of the psychotic patient must do in witnessing psychotic reality. The witness looks for any indication of this capacity. Dr. Roth's patient stuck his tongue out. A playful gesture using an object in reality, the tongue that elicited a response.

The witness must become a transitional object, at first, in reality. The witness is both found and invented. The witness is invented by the need in the patient and by their use of the witness and the role the witness has for them. To be useful, the witness must respect the patient's transitional use of the witness, both as yours and theirs. It is this relationship that Winnicott called the transitional relationship. It was the use of an object in reality (cite) for emotional growth and development in a creative-fantasy-reality mixing. Winnicott found its adult equivalence in imagination, in art, in fiction, in culture. It is also in relationships. One of the crucial features of the transitional object for Winnicott was its use as a catalyst in the growth and development of the experience of the self.

Transitions in the experience of the body become transitions in relationships with the body, and because of this, the body can be a transitional object. Such physical body transitions, from one stage of physical growth and development to another or from one state change to another, catalyze transitions in growth and development of the self. The body is a transitional catalytic object, especially during periods of rapid physical change like adolescence, sex (Marcus, 2023), and other physiologic functions, but also in illness.

When the transitional use of the body is flooded by the experience of illness, catastrophe emotions like fear and dread result. The transitional object experience with a sick body is a transitional experience that may be filled with anxious dread. Then, the transitional space is obliterated by a feared reality. It can be frightening and overwhelming and can cause an anxious stalemate in adaptation and psychological growth. A non-ill transitional object is therefore necessary.

The non-ill transitional object is the need the witness supplies. A caregiver who accompanies and witnesses this process becomes part of the transitional object process and can change the use of this physical illness experience into its use for growth and development of the self. The witness of medical illness in the patient must contain anxiety, fear, despair, paranoid mixtures of anger and fear, about the real illness. But this containment can also reinforce the boundary between the illness and the self.

With psychotic patients, the witness must contain the condensation without being able to reinforce boundaries. The witness for a psychotic patient must be able to build a mental space midway between the patient's reality experience and their psychotic reality experience by maintaining this capacity in the witness and in their witnessing.

When the psychotic condensation must be the transitional object experience for the patient, catastrophic feelings result, because reality is both contaminated by emotional experience and dominates the transitional experience so that it is obliterated as a creative capacity and as a growth potential. Nothing new can happen. It is in a psychotic status nascendi.

The witness must empathize with this and disclaim it at the same time. This is an internal experience in the witness. The care giving witness must be able to tolerate, contain, metabolize, and help the patient use this anxious dread by reinforcing reality boundaries and thus keeping hope alive. This hope exists in its greatest intensity in the transitional object experience which, in the very ill, must be externalized first in the witness. The hope is that the psychotic reality is not real.

Once the function is externalized, and taken into the witness, perhaps then the patient's self-experience of the witness can include a transitional experience, where the psychosis is used both as reality fact and as a plaything. In understanding the emotional significance of and within the psychotic condensation, there becomes an understanding that the psychotic condensation has an emotional significance, and thereby perhaps can appear a transitional relationship to it. It is perhaps ideally suited for this because the psychotic condensation is experienced as both real and meaningful symbolic, that is to say – invented!

Winnicott's genius is revealed with his observation that the transitional object is at first an object. So is the psychotic condensation. So is the witness. Both the teddy bear and the psychotic condensation are experienced as reality objects. The child can use the teddy bear as a symbolic representation for imaginative play. Later, transitional objects can be purely imaginary, in fantasy.

The witness must help the patient with psychosis do the same thing with their psychotic condensation (Garrett, 2019). Only then can the integrity of the self be reestablished and maintained. Only then can something new be synthesized; a new experience of the self. It happens first in the witness and then in the witnessing relationship, and then in the patient independently.

In summary, witnessing works if it catalyzes, creates, and conserves a container function of a specific type. It is the container of a transitional object and transitional process, hence, a catalyst to the synthesizing function of the self, a growth and development function of the self, in a protected relationship called witnessing.

Witnessing with a psychotic patient requires the ability for empathy in a transitional zone midway between the witness feelings about reality and the patient's feelings about reality; midway between ordinary reality and psychotic reality.

This type of witnessing with a psychotic patient requires not just an empathic attunement but an ability to experience that attunement in reality. The witness psychotherapist must feel is they are an object in reality with the patient.

To be an object in reality does not mean to be the real you, whatever that means, or in a real relationship with the patient, whatever that means. It means experiencing yourself with the patient in ordinary reality (Winnicott, 1971). You relate to the psychotic patient from a stance of your feeling that the two of you are in an ordinary reality experience. Later, transitional objects can be purely imaginary; in fantasy.

Not all of us can do it. Those who can are to be appreciated. Dr. Roth is one of them. He acted in the context of an ordinary reality experience. This allowed him to recognize, in contrast, that the tongue gesture was play. Play occurs in a transitional space but with an object in reality. He recognizes the capacity in the psychotic patient that will perhaps be an open vehicle for treatment. He then aprichiates it. He then might even participate in it. Sticking out his tongue as a response, with a smile. It is this kind of receptivity and flexibility within ordinary reality that is a requirement of work with psychotic patients.

This is because a delusion is an in reality experience. It is frozen and without reality testing. This means the capacity to see it as anything other than a reality experience is gone. But around each delusion and hallucination is an associated penumbra of experience about which reality testing is potentially there. That is the reality fantasy mix potential. The tongue gesture was an invitation into that space, which Dr. Roth understood and accepted. That is why the conversation immediately progressed to who said what to whom. I believe the patient was alluding to his auditory hallucinations in which he was told to say and do things. The patient was remarking that this tongue gesture he was not told to do. This was voluntary. This came from the real him, not from the psychotic him. A spontaneous gesture from the nonpsychotic real him. A further huge step was taken when the patient asks if Dr. Roth was told to stick his tongue out or what to say. This allows Dr. Roth to say no he was not told what to do or say. Thus was Dr. Roth able to disclaim psychotic reality and stand firmly in ordinary reality. The patient was then able to have a self-experience of agency in nonpsychotic reality. The patient said I wasn't told to do or say this either. This was a first step toward freeing the self from the psychotic part. This is what is meant by a real relationship with a psychotic patient; it means a relationship in reality. If it is purely an emotional transference relationship, the danger is that it will be a psychotic transference.

With psychotic patients, we are asked to do something difficult, to empathize with, and to understand their psychotic reality experience. We are asked to contain in our reality experience of the patient, their psychotic reality experience. It requires a calm certainty about reality at the same moment of empathic holding of another's psychotic reality. It is not easy. It does not immediately produce a change. It is why witness is a better term for our work, especially in the beginning when they don't first recognize their psychosis as an illness so our work is not as a therapist but as a witness. Our goal is to be able to tolerate the experience. It is the first step in helping them tolerate it.

If the patient knows that you feel it, the patient will have been witnessed. Their empathy for your empathy of them helps them with their empathy for you where they find empathy for themselves. This back-and-forth requires yourself in reality. This can be the first step in them of an observing ego about reality and therefore about their psychosis. It starts with the pathway of empathizing with the suffering to them their psychosis is causing and which you are witnessing. It helps them sanctify their experience of their suffering by psychosis as a meaning event not requiring the sanctification of psychotic reality. Being the real you in your witness function does not require self-exposure of private areas of yourself. It involves the ability to feel the real you and the real them, both of you together, in ordinary reality. It is a give and take about reality, not about you.

This witnessing process can be used for a new compromise synthesis in the self's relationship to the psychosis. New relationships require new syntheses both of the person to the other and of the person to themselves. Synthesis itself is a type of mastery and control, first of emotion, then of meaning of fact, via the context of fact, and then of the change in self-experience of the fact. The witness becomes part of that context and provides the possibility for a new relationship of the psychotic person to the witness and therefore to the witness' view of reality, and therefore to reality itself and therefore helps the patient realistically view their own psychosis. This might then proceed to a de-condensation of the psychotic experience.

Because being the witness to suffering creates our own suffering, the witness has also the need to be witnessed. This requires in us a growth and development capacity for self-witness and for our use of the witness experience. The suffering of another can become a transitional object for us in our own growth as witnesses. This transitional object must occur in relationship to ourselves as well as in our relationship to the patient. Dr. Roth does that when he enjoys sticking his tongue out. Self-witnessing is a transitional growth process with its own phases of professional growth and development.

In the beginning, the transitional object for the witness tends to be the patient's illness. With experience that becomes the patient themselves and their suffering. Strengthening the witness function is the witness' ego ideal; the professional, craft ideal. This ideal consolidates and is molded during training and it is one reason we call it training rather than education. This professional ego ideal has its own growth and development sequence but hopefully it neither rigidifies, causing robotic applications of preformed interactions, nor stagnates causing burnout. This slowly evolving ego ideal continues to grow and change and to provide new capacities for generative empathy as we ourselves grow in experience of mastery and of effective goodness in our profession.

Concurrent with this and development of the ego ideal are the stages of growth of therapeutic empathy (Marcus, 2003). These stages change from empathic identity, to empathic dis-identity, to empathic hesitancy that is goal directed, to empathic resonance that is at first externally goal directed and with further growth becomes also internally goal directed. In work with psychotic patients, progressive changes in empathy capacity and the ego ideal need a progressive ability to focus on the transitional experience of healthy reality and on the processes rather than the facts, and on the future rather than the present. It also crucially focuses on our ability to help rather than their inability to receive help. This is where a mature professional ego ideal is really needed.

From the transitional treatment process comes a new synthesis about the person, their life, their historical events, their stressors and traumas, their emotional development, and their emotional adaptation, of which the psychotic condensation is one type. A story ties together the facts with the emotional significance of the facts.

There is a relationship between the illness history, the life history, and the emotional history. It can be found in the relationship among them which we call story. The psychotic illness forms a psychotic story and is psychotic only because it is experienced in reality experience with the loss of reality testing. But all story is a record of the links between what happens and how it makes people feel about themselves because of those happenings. This then affects the sequential relationship of meanings in what happens. Delusions and hallucinations are highly condensed, psychotic stories.

People do and don't knit together stories in people-specific ways forming a pattern of doing so and not doing so that is their story style, their personality. This is one relationship of personality to psychosis. It isn't the causal relationship. It is the adaptive relationship. Everyone has knitting, failures to knit, and un-ravelings that are characteristic. We say it is an aspect of personality. This should be recognized as part of the material medica of care giving. Seeing the pattern can help the witness help the patient see that pattern and take their next step of mastering this process for themselves. In this way, treatment of psychosis can also be treatment of personality and result in deeper understanding and growth of the self.

In summary, therapeutic relationships like witnessing can be a transitional process in which the relationship is not only a real one but also a symbolic one. Witnessing works because relationships as well as events have symbolic meaning and become thereby signifiers of deep emotional meaning. These then take their place as perhaps nodal points in story generation and evolution. "And then I met Dr. Roth." We will have to understand, as Dr. Roth does, the therapeutic moments in the story, the nodal points, where change is possible and indicate our receptivity to it. That is what therapeutic witnessing, and all psychotherapy requires. Especially with the psychotic patient. Spontaneously responding to the spontaneous gesture. Stick your tongue out.

References

Bion, W. R. (1970) Container and Contained. In *Attention & Interpretation*. Exeter: Wheaton & Co, ch. 7, pp. 72–82.

Garrett, M. (2019) *Psychotherapy for Psychosis: Integrating Cognitive, Behavioral, and Psychodynamic Treatment*. New York and London: The Guilford Press.

Marcus, E. (2003) Medical Student Dreams about Medical School: The Unconscious Developmental Process of Becoming a Physician. *The International Journal of Psychoanalysis* 84:367–386.

Marcus, E. (2017) *Psychosis and Near Psychosis: Ego Function, Symbol Structure, Treatment*. London and New York: Routledge.

Marcus, E. (2023) *Modern Ego Psychology and Human Sexual Experience: The Meaning of Treatment*. London and New York: Routledge.

Miriam-Webster' Dictionary. Copywrite (2024) Springfield Mass.

Poland, W. (2000) The Analyst's Witnessing and Otherness. *Journal of the American Psychoanalytic Association* 48:17–34.

Schafer, R. (1959) Generative Empathy in the Treatment Situation. *The Psychoanalytic Quarterly* 28:342–373.

Winnicott, D. W. (1971a) Good Enough Mother. In *Playing and Reality*. London: Tavistock Publications, p. 10.

Winnicott, D. W. (1971b) Transitional Objects and Transitional Phenomena. In *Playing and Reality*. London: Tavistock Publications, pp. 1–25.

Winnicott, D. W. (1971c) The Use of an Object and Relating Through Identifications. In *Playing and Reality*. London: Tavistock Publications, pp. 86–94.

4 Comment on Dr. Bennett E. Roth's experiences with a psychotic young man dominated by an internal pathological organization

Paul Williams

It is always refreshing to see a beneficial outcome of humane and creative inter-action between a dedicated psychotherapist and a desperate patient sufficiently hungry for change to both recognize and make use of the offer of an authentic relationship. This form of vitality is conveyed in Dr. Roth's account in a personal way, reflecting the kind of work done with D. There is a great deal that could be said about the case from both theoretical and technical perspectives. I shall, however, confine my comment to the terrible, cruel control exerted by the internal psychotic organization in Daniel which acts perversely *in loco parentis*, ostensibly to pre-vent further damage to the ego, if necessary even at the cost of the patient's life. How this torturing creature and its manifestations come into being is relevant in the treatment of much severe disturbance. I have come to understand the orchestrating activity at the heart of internal pathological organizations as being a response to a catastrophic failure in infancy of containment of projections of overwhelming affective and sensorial experiences. The rudimentary building blocks of ego forma-tion are, as a result, not formed or fail to cohere due to this lack of containment and thus the infant's inability to achieve 'successful' splitting, and are projected violently into part objects and aspects of the environment. In particular, frustration and aggression are experienced as intolerable, leading to projected fantasies and parts of the mind becoming organized to produce a form of pathological contain-ment of a non-symbolized, static, and essentially psychotic kind. This pathological organization activity permeates the subject's life, influencing attitudes and behavior in all situations but with the overriding aim of preventing a repetition of the original traumatizing experience of the infant. Paradoxically, the methods used to prevent re-traumatization and protect the damaged ego can closely resemble the trauma the subject has suffered, but they are rendered effective through forms of seduction that inveigle the mind into a delusional sense of security. The ego is, essentially, brainwashed into now and forever remaining distant from people and the external world, despite its desperate need for help. Threats are made when the ego attempts to gain help from people and the external world, and this gives rise to internal oscil-lation between sadistic punishment and sexualized enticement, leading to isolation. Meanwhile, the nascent personality of the subject remains corralled and immobile, 'ensuring' the survival of the damaged ego (Williams 2014).

DOI: 10.4324/9781003427049-5

Dr. Roth was fortunate to be in circumstances in which the hospital institution, thanks in part to the collegial support he received, tolerated his unconventional approach. It is, in my opinion, vitally important that the crippled imagination of the psychotic individual be helped to engage in some form of creative, and thereby hopeful, human dialogue. This activity will be met with serious opposition by the psychosis and the pathological organization. The account of D demonstrates a profound wish to engage alongside terror and psychotic defensiveness and thus provides valuable insights into his attempts to relate in order for him to try to find his own mind. My own understanding of the sticking out of tongues and penises by both parties was that of a primitive kind of greeting that contained concrete, visceral expressions of aggression and sexuality in the service of a most basic form of recognition. When D began to talk, it was in a similarly primitive way denoting, to my mind, experiences of isolation and affective denudation where human relating should have been. The emphasis on 'Nobody' and 'Gone' (themes echoed in a brief chapter below taken from a similar but rather more disturbed individual than D) seem to denote the profound, schizoid dilemma of the psychotic patient who has no good internal object and who has had to withdraw from humanity. In place of a trustworthy object is a rudimentary and confused collation of something called nobody which seems to control D's emotional life. His contact and more alive interaction with his new therapist lead to night terrors and screaming, which I take to be a negative psychotic reaction to human contact. Dr. Roth, determined to find points of identification with D, struggles to elucidate potential symbolic inferences from D's concrete, enigmatic statements. I suspect that this determination to take D seriously had a profound effect on him: a vital psychoanalytic 'third' was now engaged, something that had previously been missing. The incident with the occupational therapist is particularly sad but instructive in that it reveals how easily the power of psychosis can be underestimated in patients. If the clay figure of a large beaked bird's head on a bear-like frame with alligator feet and claws did have symbolic connections to D's mother in his unconscious, then to encourage D to smash this figure could unfortunately have the effect of re-traumatizing D who in all likelihood feels himself to be responsible for his mother's troubles and his own infantile trauma. A repetition of this murder of the mother sends D into a catatonic withdrawal.

When Dr. Roth makes an attempt to stand up to 'Nobody', it has the effect of making D smile and to reply: 'Nobody will get you', which I took to be a statement of fear on D's part. By resorting to a form of omnipotence (a battle of 'Gods' – Dr. Roth vs. Nobody), the omnipotence of the psychotic organization was inflamed within D who, perhaps smiling to conceal his anxiety, warns Dr. Roth of his impending fate if he continues to challenge the psychosis directly. We can't talk a person out of psychosis: the best we can do is to create a triangle in which two nonpsychotic minds engage in the deepest conversation possible around what it feels like to be insane. I take the various voices and representations of figures and part objects in D to be variations of the psychosis driving the pathological organization. Infantile projections of uncontained experiences coexist in a wilderness as projected 'beta' elements, in a jarring and un-integrated way producing emotional violence and conflict because integration of experiences feels impossible. In my experience, this can be a reason why statements in psychosis can contain more than one meaning. 'Be right back' is an example provided by D. This can be a reassurance; it can be an expression of undefeated omnipotence; and it can be a hint of a sane communication denoting the distance D has to remain from objects. There are likely to be many more meanings than these speculative associations that Dr. Roth discovered in his study of D's use of language.

The event in which Dr. Roth took Daniel outside the ward seems to me to be very important in that it was an attempt to face the external world in a humane way, not least by the powerful symbolism of linking of arms that may have helped generate a form of equality and connectedness that D could hold onto. Clinging to the bottle of soda made me wonder about D's precarious clinging to life, and the dead seagull that produced so much alarm may have been the D who died emotionally in infancy. There being no such thing as death in the unconscious, D is horrified to see the seagull and engages in a primitive warding off of death, at least now not alone. The question of psychosis and death in the personality is insufficiently explored in the psychoanalytic literature. The condition of soul murder (evident in the chapter below) is closely allied, in my view, to the impact of psychosis on the infant personality. It remains to be discovered to what extent psychosis in infancy has a relationship with soul murder, and if so of what kind. Abuse and emotional neglect are principal characteristics of soul murder, and not all infants who become psychotic suffer in this way. At the same time, psychosis destroys personality functioning and development in ways that can be similar to experiences of soul murder: differentiating the two is an important matter. What occurs in soul murder seems to me to be linked with Winnicott's understanding of the need for protection of the inviolable nature of the 'isolate' which is the nearest thing to the soul mentioned by Winnicott (1966). Exposure and damage to the isolate seem, in some people, to vitiate the development or recovery of inherent object seeking and object relating capacities. This does not appear to be the case with D, although the account does not make this entirely clear. On the basis of the clinical changes reported, the youth and plasticity of D's mind still permit an eagerness to engage despite his severe illness and catatonic withdrawal. For soul murder to eventuate it may be that wholesale destruction or absence of any good internal object relating experience is necessary. This may contribute to psychosis, and if so the two require careful study and each needs to be thought about in somewhat different, albeit related, terms.

References

Williams, P. (2014). Orientations of Psychotic Activity in Defensive Pathological Organizations. *The International Journal of Psychoanalysis* 95(3):423–440.

Winnicott, D. W. (1963) Communicating and Not Communicating Leading to a Study of Certain Opposites. In *The Maturational Processes and the Facilitating Environment: Studies in the Theory of Emotional Development.* London: The International Psycho-Analytic Library.

5 Discussion of Dr. Bennett E. Roth's case of a catatonic boy

Annie Reiner

Bion wrote a significant amount regarding language in his later years, about how we communicate both with our patients and our colleagues. I have recently explored his ideas about the limitations of a verbal language that is essentially derived from our sense-based experiences of the physical world, but which we then have to try to apply to the infinite, unconscious, metaphysical realm of the mind, that Bion called "O" (Reiner, 2022). I think the mystery of that invisible mind is reflected in some of the struggles that Dr. Roth's patient, D, grapples with, and which I will discuss later in relation to D's "No body," and the invisible Voice.

I should explain that I am using the term "mind" as Bion used it, not as is commonly used to reflect intellectual or ego functions, but as synonymous with one's self, one's personality, or spirit – one's fundamental being. This is of central importance to my comments about this case, which reflect Bion's ideas about what constitutes a mind, and what contributes to its development, or the lack of development, of a mind or self. This fundamental idea is based on Bion's early theories of thinking, where he posits that the mother's capacity for reverie facilitates her ability to experience, contain, and dream the infant's emotional experiences, which serves as a model for the child's own eventual ability to feel and contain his or her own feelings. These feelings can then be digested and processed as thoughts. Without this kind of emotional connection with the mother's mind, the development of the child's mind – with its capacities to feel and think – is obstructed.

I should also preface my response to this chapter by saying that my thoughts about D are conjectures and educated guesses, since I have never actually met the patient. But Bion recommended that even in one's own sessions, one needs to engage in what he called, "science fictions," or "imaginative conjectures." This enables one to use one's imaginations to contact the patient's imagination, his or her unconscious and primitive proto-mental states of mind. This contrast with relying on what one already knows, one's theories, which are intellectual and tend to engage the patient's intellect, rather than the full emotional presence of the patient. These conjectures are not so different than discussions we have with colleagues or students in any case conference, or in cases one supervises, because as Bion often reminded everyone, only the patient and the

DOI: 10.4324/9781003427049-6

analyst (or therapist) are actually present to experience each other. And yet even for them, their interaction may feel like the stuff of dreams, difficult to grasp, since what happens in these interchanges of inner life between two people, are complex, invisible, and impressionistic at best.

In short, my conjectures are not meant to challenge what Dr. Roth did or said, but are responses to the case from my own perspective. They are my dreams about Daniel's unconscious dreams that may be useful in thinking about his state of mind, with the hope of learning something more about it. Grotstein writes that whether or not a patient reports a dream, each session can itself be taken as a dream – a product of his unconscious – for analytic purposes. I'm suggesting that we can treat the events of Daniels sessions this way, to understand more about his inner experiences.

About our use of language in clinical work, Bion wrote, "In psychoanalysis we have to manufacture our means of communication while we are communicating" (Bion, 1975, p. 39). This idea seems relevant to Dr. Roth's experience with this case. Daniel presented here with some characteristic behaviors of catatonia – rigid, repetitive, and purposeless actions – and he was verbally uncommunicative, a self-imposed silence that his therapist managed to penetrate before too long. This progress in the early sessions makes a very good case for why Bion so often stressed the need for therapists and analysts to stop relying on theories, including his, so we could feel and think for ourselves about the specific, living person in front of us. This was part of Bion's (1967) advice for the analyst to suspend his memory (what one already knows in the past) and his desire (one's hopes for the future), in order to make real emotional contact. This living language of psychoanalysis is born of the moment, in a particular relationship to a particular patient on a particular day. Our theories, he cautioned, were of precious little use to the patient, like intellectual relics to be examined or admired, but which could not penetrate to a vital, emotional, and unknown part of the patient. Likewise, our reliance on "experts" like one's analyst or teachers, created an opaque, impenetrable obstacle. In the session, he said, "There is no one to fall back on but yourself" (Bion, 1977). It is a lonely place, as one senses in Dr. Roth's early, silent sessions with this silent adolescent who moved oddly, and marched stiffly "like a toy soldier."

Suspension of memory, desire, and understanding

Bion's (1967, 1970) central clinical idea about the analyst's need to suspend memory, desire, and understanding while in session with the patient is an aspect of this idea that only the therapist was in a position to speak meaningfully to the patient. For instance, there is nothing in psychoanalytic theory that suggests that the analyst or therapist should respond to a patient who sticks out his tongue, by sticking out one's own tongue. And yet at the moment it happened, sticking out his tongue was perhaps the best, or only, "language" that Daniel had at his disposal. Though its meaning may not have been clear, Dr. Roth was able to "reply" to Daniel's communication in a way that seemed meaningful to Daniel. Dr. Roth admits that he let his mind wander, "preoccupied with my own phantasies" (p. 4), which at times can be very useful, although it could also become a state of detachment in which two people are left there, unable to connect to each other. Its usefulness relates to the state of mind that Freud (1912) described as "evenly hovering attention," which facilitates the analyst's capacity for open-mindedness and intuition. This is a similar state of mind to Bion (1970) described as a waking-dream state that facilitated contact with what he called "O," which he viewed as the central psychoanalytic perspective. Both of these states may seem like, but are vastly different from, the detachment of succumbing to one's own inner world. But it is a fine line, and Bion (1978) points out that the difference is hard to explain, calling O, "a peculiar state of mind . . . [where] the margin between being consciously awake . . . and being asleep, is extremely small" (p. 41). If one succumbs to sleep, that is going too far, but if one is hyper-awake, one cannot access the dream-like, and deeply intuitive state. Dream states are important to the capacity to think. Thinking is dependent on access to dream states that Bion called "alpha function" (p.), which are important in the mother and infant, and in the analyst and analysand. This is why Grotstein (2007) said, "Thinking itself is, according to Bion, is essentially unconscious" (p. 47).

Developing more sophisticated uses of one's intuition depends on that waking-dream state, but this typically takes many years to cultivate. So what is one to do as a young therapist faced with an enigmatic patient like D? In this case, Dr. Roth's ability to relax and give over to his phantasies proved very useful, for what may have seemed random, really was not. As he explained, seeing D stick out his tongue evoked an association to baby-sitting his nephews, where one might feel more comfortable being playful, and sticking out his tongue certainly had that playful quality. Winnicott's ideas of play are not unlike Bion's ideas of the importance of dreaming, both of which involve unconscious thought processes. Winnicott (1971) called play essential for psychotherapy, saying, "If the therapist cannot play, then he is not suitable for the work" (p. 54). He described play as the essence of creativity and wrote, "Creative apperception . . . makes the person feel that life is worth living" (ibid., p. 65). I think, this describes D's feeling in that session, having reacted to Dr. Roth's sticking out his tongue as an authentic, playful, and communicative gesture, and his reaction was dramatic – he spoke. It seemed to engage in this boy what I would call "hope," for Dr. Roth's reaction to D born in part of his thought about his young nephews, was appropriate to a small child or baby. Mirroring back Daniel's behavior seemed to give him a sense that he existed, for he could see evidence of his existence in his therapist's face. It was real and spontaneous, not theoretical.

It seems to me that words were already tainted by meaninglessness for this boy who, for the most part, exists at a very primitive, pre-verbal level of emotional development. Dr. Roth's visual response aroused his interest and his curiosity at that level, as it would in a very small infant. Although D learned how to speak, like most children, it does not mean that it is meaningful for all children, especially if his real self or mind had not yet developed. But in this case, D not only speaks, he says something meaningful, although most likely neither he nor Dr. Roth is at that moment aware of its meaning. And so he asks his therapist, "Who told you to do that?" (p. 4)

One gets the sense that in this moment D is astonished by the possibility that this man he is with may actually know or care that he exists, for he reacted to him in a real way. D's question, however, also seems to embody his disbelief in the possibility that such a thing exists as someone who can react to him, and not in a rigid way dictated by rules he learned to obey but does not understand. Babies instinctively "understand" meaningful connection, for it underlies the physiological instinct for attachment that helps insure their survival, but if the infant's instinctual need meets with an anxious, depressed, or otherwise emotionally detached mother, that child begins to *unlearn* the basic and essential á priori knowledge of attachment that presages love. I have seen so many patients who were never authentically understood or emotionally noticed by their parents, parents who may have had good intentions, but who themselves lacked the capacity for emotional attachment. These patients never had the opportunity to develop a "voice" of their own, to know what they thought or felt, or express it, for they had never been heard, and one can imagine that Daniel similarly got used to hearing and saying things that were not authentic. Such children learn to speak in the voice of what Winnicott (1965) called the False Self, which "organizes the suicide" of the true self (p. 143). This mental/emotional death leaves a self unable to develop a real self.

For D, this moment of connection and hope were mixed, as I said, with wariness and confusion, for it was unfamiliar. Someone had "spoken" to him, however, which seemed to create in him enough interest and curiosity to be moved to reply. When Dr. Roth repeats Daniel's question – "Who told you to do that?" – D says, "Nobody told me." This evoked a meaningful subject, an unconscious one and so one that was not easily recognizable. It seemed to me to indicate that what D is dealing with is the absence of a self that can feel, think, or exist. We might read that as "Nobody told me to stick out my tongue, I did it all on my own," but we might also read it as "Somebody who isn't really anybody told me to stick out my tongue." Is this the same Nobody that moves so rigidly because he is a no-body that does not recognize his body as part of his self? As Dr. Roth says, he "marches" everywhere, stiff, rigid, disembodied, like No body. It has the feeling of someone in the Army, following rigid rules by submerging anything spontaneous or personal, and I would guess that this need to follow orders, perhaps from a torturous, primitive superego, may reflect the absence of a mind that knows anything about what to do or what has meaning. I thought the ray of hope in this interchange was that perhaps D was not completely Nobody, a hope that if he had someone who could see him, and interact with him at his level, then perhaps he did exist.

Still, it can be terrifying suddenly to have one's existence noticed, for he had also clearly worked very hard to protect himself from any kind of contact or feeling. Perhaps it was this hint of realness that gave rise to the screams and night terrors that D was soon reported to have had. He had been given the diagnosis of catatonia, but we know that diagnoses overlap, and there are certainly elements of autism in this boy, including the painful states of nonexistence and nothingness, of being No body. The terror of beginning to be makes it evident that being No-body is paradoxically both the problem and the cure.

We speak of languages as "tongues," and the language between D and Dr. Roth was one where the tongue itself did the speaking. While it spoke in movement rather than sound or words, it is a language, nonetheless, and clearly a powerful one, since it gave him, if only for a moment, that sense that he existed in the face or being of the other.

Nobody or No body?

Is "No body" an individual who has no identity, no self, or is it an individual with no physical body? While it is unclear what D means, perhaps he means both. Does one physically exist without a metaphysical mind that identifies his body as part of his self? Although this sounds like a philosophical question far beyond the primitive mental level at which D seems to operate, autistic children do experience the feeling of being nothing and nobody, a feeling of nonexistence. It is not that they, or D, have the capacity to think this, or to know what this terrifying feeling is, but the terror is real. For such patients, we must first help them to develop a mind to feel its feelings. Dr. Roth's first intuitive impulse to mirror D sticking out his tongue was one example of this sort of mirroring containment of a part of D's experience. I would not be surprised if on a deeply unconscious level, it was an expression of an idea that there was something wrong with his tongue, that is, with his capacity for language, communication, and thought, as well as the earlier uses of his tongue in nursing, and the confusion between his self (tongue) and his mother (nipple). It is the mother's reverie that gives her an experience of her infant's feelings, so the infant can begin to recognize those feelings as parts of him. The analyst needs to be able to descend into these often-terrifying places of nonbeing to learn more about where the patient is. One may then be in a position to help him to think about experiences that he had no other way to know about, and no way to express except in these cryptic and rigid ways.

Voice with No-body

In a later session, Dr. Roth came to think that No-body was a Voice with no body that Daniel hears, that is, a disembodied Voice. We could also say it is a voice he cannot see, and whose origins are unknown. I began to think that from the perspective of the metaphysical mind described by Bion, the "voice" may represent Daniel's invisible and unknown thoughts/feelings whose origins are equally invisible and unknown to him. Very young infants do not know what feelings are, or even that they are parts of oneself. For instance, a feeling of hunger is new for the infant, and may be interpreted as some sort of unknown attack by a dangerous monster, a monster of his own fear, frustration, and hatred, perhaps. Primitive feelings, what Bion calls the psychotic parts of the personality, can in fact develop into psychosis, without a parent able to allay some of these imaginative, but false theories.

I saw evidence for these ideas and their link to language in Daniel's image, or voice, of a "very large parakeet that spoke without its mouth moving" (p. 11). Perhaps this parakeet fits in with the idea of No body, a disembodied voice that can only parrot back someone else's language without really knowing what he is saying, or why, and without really knowing what anyone else is really saying either, or why. Grown-ups mouths may be moving but he cannot understand that they have meaning. It reflects a fundamental distrust of language, including his own, that may in part explain his choice to be silent.

Babies learn to talk by parroting the sounds they hear, but if emotional connection is compromised in the relationship between mother and infant, children may fail to develop the capacity for a mind that can *use that* language in meaningful ways, to communicate or to think. This No-body, or No-baby, may still learn to speak but the language is more like echolalia than meaningful speech, a debased or false language of a false self.

We also later learn of D's having decapitated his mother's parakeet, which provides possible evidence that these feelings are related to feelings about his mother. Did he decapitate her? Was she already "decapitated," in the sense of not being able to use her head/mind to connect with her son? Had he then also wanted to find a way to express that this had decapitated him?

Summary and conclusions

Bion redefined what we mean by a "mind." Meltzer (1984) described how both Freud and Klein assumed the existence of a mind that could already think about and respond to what we say, while Bion's idea of a mind is of a mental *potential* that either develops in the infant's relationship to the mother, or it does not. It led Bion to this thought about whether the human mind – the very focus of our work – exists at all.

> Let us hope that such a thing as a mind, a personality, a character exists, and that we are not just talking about nothing.
>
> (Bion, 1978, p. 317)

Bion gives voice here to the mystery at the heart of psychoanalytic inquiry, namely a mind/self/personality whose existence is improvable through sensory means. While Bion himself did believe in the existence of this enigmatic mind, he did not think it was something analysts had agreed upon. Inherent in Bion's idea is the need to determine with any patient whether they are mentally present or not. It is certainly relevant to D's experience, but it is also a question that is applicable to many high-functioning, neurotic patients. At the end of his chapter about D, Dr. Roth bravely asks, "What role did my honest ignorance play in his treatment." I would say that it was a big one, but a very useful one. Bion (1977) often advised us to make peace with our ignorance, to focus less on answers and more on questions. If we can bear our ignorance, we might stimulate our capacity to be curious about what we don't know, to be open to something new, a new thought, or like Dr. Roth's unexpected gesture, which seemed to allow D to open up as well.

In my clinical seminar with Bion, he one day asked us, "What language is this patient speaking?" We did not know what he meant, but it opened our minds to the idea that there is more to language than the lexical or syntactic meaning. I think the question has great meaning in this case, for while children learn the language of their families and cultures, this does not mean, as we see with D, that anybody has learned *his* language. Perhaps the "nobody" he says is gone, is D, for if he could never develop into "somebody," that somebody may have been replaced by the nobody of a false self – with neither a body nor a mind. If another living somebody who could hear his emotional language did not see the somebody he might have been, there can be no self. So I think that Dr. Roth's instinctual impulse to engage in a different kind of physical language, was the start of a primitive language more appropriate to Daniel's actual pre-verbal, and proto-mental level of development.

References

Bion, W. R. (1967) Notes on Memory and Desire. In *Cogitations*. London: Karnac, pp. 380–385.

Bion, W. R. (1970) *Attention and Interpretation*. London: Karnac.

Bion, W. R. (1975) Bion (1977) *Private Clinical Seminar*. Los Angeles: Bion's Home.

Bion, W. R. (1978) *Four Discussion with W. R. Bion*. Perthshire, Scotland: Cluny Press.

Freud, S. (1912) Freud, S. 'Recommendations to Physicians Practising Psychoanalysis', S.E., 12. London: Hogarth Press.

Grotstein, J. (2007) *A Beam of Intense Darkness*. London: Karnac.

Meltzer, D. (1984) The Relation of Dreaming to Learning from Experience in Patient and Analyst. In *Dream Life: A Re-examination of the Psycho-analytical Theory and Technique*. Strath Tay, Perthshire: Clunie Press.

Reiner, A. (2022) Limitations of Language in the Psychic Realm. In A. Reiner (ed.) *W. R. Bion's Theories of Mind: A Contemporary Introduction*. London: Routledge, pp. 4–14.

Winnicott, D. W. (1965) *The Maturational Processes and the Facilitating Environment*. London: Karnac.

Winnicott, D. W. (1971) *Playing & Reality*. London: Karnac.

6 Comment on Dr. Bennett E. Roth's experiences with a catatonic psychotic boy

Technical challenges of working with the Psychotic and the nonpsychotic part

Karyn Todes

In his final sentence of the paper, Dr. Roth asked himself, "What role did my honest ignorance play in his treatment? Dr. Roth talks to his patient from "inside out," using his intuition and his own willingness to initiate a dialogue with D, in a manner that is not schooled and free from rigidity. In this sense from the outset his position is polar opposite to his patient who he describes as rigid. These polar opposites demonstrate two different ways of being. D is closed down and projecting massively from his internal world. He did not have a thinking apparatus, where as Dr. Roth has a thinking apparatus, is open minded, lost, and trying to take in the experience of his patient.

The analytic work begins, before a sound has been uttered by D or his analyst. It seems less important that Dr. Roth doesn't know what to make of his thoughts yet, and is not sure how to technically proceed. Rather he is willing to wait for the moment he receives something in his mind. In this sense, Dr. Roth demonstrates an analytic stance/model when working with a psychotic patient. Bion's notion of the "unrepresented unconscious" and the analysts expanding capacity to listen beyond the words (and in this patient to the almost non-existent narrative, and psychotic process) is central.

D's thinking apparatus is fragmented, split broken, and seemingly incomprehensible. In the introduction, and throughout the narrative, Dr. Roth alludes to the internal voices that he thinks exist in D's mind. Dr. Roth relays that D set his house on fire, leaving the reader with phantasies about where the fire is in D who is catatonic. D's lack of speech hoses down the level of destructiveness that might exist in this psychotic patient. Is the fire the agent of destruction of D's inner world, resulting in his disintegrated ego? There must have been a psychotic idea that D was going to be set on fire or killed, or somebody was threatening him, so he had to try kill them before they killed him. Fire is directed to his psychotic enemies or assailants, but is also directed toward D himself – toward his nonpsychotic part, or his sane wishes. In setting his house on fire, he is possibly both killing himself and killing others simultaneously. It is unlikely there was any containment of his feelings from the time he was

DOI: 10.4324/9781003427049-7

an infant. With this in mind, D might have been catatonic and mute to protect everyone including himself, from himself.

Dr. Roth, in attending to his own emotional response to his patient, throughout the work, potentially carries parts of his patient projected into him, about which D is oblivious. Using Dr. Roth's own body and mind, he responds to this nonsensical, stiff, confusing state he is thrust into by his patient. He assumes, for example, a boxing stance on one occasion, perhaps an action revealing something that cannot be thought about or felt yet by either Dr. Roth nor D.

The analyst worries that he will be "laughed at," mocked by his colleagues in the hospital. I am reminded of it, toward the end of the psychotherapy when the chief psychiatrist acts with suspicion looking oddly at Dr. Roth, mistrusting B. Roth's intervention. Who, does this suspicious mocking voice represent, and is it an aspect of the psychotic part of D? Perhaps, B. Roth is observing in himself, this part of D that unknowingly mocks D. There is always a nonpsychotic part, an analyst is trying to find in treatment of a psychotic patient, and Dr. V who is supportive of the work, and Dr. Roth seem to represent this part of the patient. The nonpsychotic part is felt "outside" in others, not "inside" the patient, and gives the analyst access to thinking without being destroyed. In this way, the presence, of a nonpsychotic part offers some hope that the work of human emotional engagement might be a little possible.

The hospital was a very conventional one. Perhaps, it seemed to represent the infectious quality of shame people feel about mental illness. Being made to feel disturbed by D or B. Roth's interactions with D might have been a very troubling experience for the staff. Dr's are faced with their own craziness when presented with psychotic patients. Massive projective identification affects the staff, who often, in fear of being driven mad, want to quiet or lock patients up, sometimes because of the impact patients have on staff. Perhaps even the chief psychiatrist's respectability and anxiety about becoming too associated with disturbing behavior is because of the impact on him, his reputation and the institutions reputation, resulted in his trying to shut things down. I was struck by the speed at which the Director of psychiatry used his authority to control B. Roth, who challenged the system by tolerating and entering into D's insane world. Psychosis also poses a problem for institutions. Do we shut it down or tolerate it? B. Roth's material reveals how the psychotic process run through every layer of the system as the psychotic bits are being projected outward, and psychosis is infectious.

Ben Roth comments that he himself wonders if when D said "he was blind," whether D thought that Ben Roth could not see him because he was "nowhere." That was a delusion in which the true self was withdrawn. In D's mind, nobody could see him and he was protected. D also could not see the projection he was making of his own incapacity to see his own problem. When he is "gone," he feels gratified and safe, but he can't see that he is blinding himself to the desperate situation he is in. He lacks alpha function, so he needs to keep projecting in an analytic relationship until he is free of enough of his projections so as to allow himself to see, that the analyst might see him and that the beginnings of visibility might take place. Everything D is experiencing is being pushed out of his mind. Ben Roth has to receive it, no matter how confusing it is, and once that happens and there is progressive containment, the projections will lessen, and beta elements can be returned to D in a more palatable form.

A parallel process seems evident, as Ben Roth makes the decision not to confide in any colleagues at the hospital as to the real nature of the interaction with D after the sessions. In keeping it secret, and not telling anybody, Roth (as analyst) continues to not be seen, and to not have his patient seen either. This part of D that remains "no where" perhaps gets enacted. Analytic work exposes mental pain rather than concealing or suppressing it. Perhaps D might have also frightened Dr. Roth who might not at that time, have felt he would be contained by his colleagues, given the extent of D's disturbance. Dr. Roth may have been infected by D (as might the director later on). To be "gone," to be "no where," would mean that he had experienced some impingement on the "isolate" inside him (Winnicott, 2016). His defenses have been stripped and he is barely a person. D has a very rudimentary fragmented true self that has never cohered, and he has never developed enough to have an adequate false self. In a state of "gone," the isolate must help the baby survive by going deeper into hiding and that way there is a chance of life.

In the start of their encounter Ben Roth's thoughts wonder off to vacations and holidays. Remaining in the vicinity of the awful unthinkable state of "no body" during the beginning sessions is difficult to tolerate, relentless, and inescapable. Roth wonders to himself how he might find a different job. Perhaps unconsciously it is to do with the dread at that moment of working with D. Alternatively, having a phantasy about a holiday or a different job, might not only be despairing, it might also represent a hope for an escape. Was Roth experiencing in himself the hope for D that D was unable to tolerate? D's situation was impossible in D's mind. Perhaps projection of this hope into Roth, was the way D communicated his desires and wishes, alongside his insane bits. Perhaps D needed to escape from hope to hate, as hate might have felt better to him then hope. Hope might have been seen by D to be a source of death.

When D starts to speak, the dialogue between Ben Roth and D has the quality of an "echo," a voice that boomerangs back and forth between them, an "it" bouncing upon the rim of a void. Without a tongue one cannot speak, and it is as if in presenting his tongue to Roth, D lets something out, only to put it back inside again. Roth then, using his reverie, recalls an emotional connection that he has with his nephews and draws on the reverie responding back with the use of his own tongue. It seems Roth is acutely aware of the infantile aspect of D, via his mouth, the first organ a baby uses to suck and latch on so as to feed. This creative act of the analyst appears to give rise to the first words D uttered. The tongue is a tongue of a young man and an infant, perhaps a form of hello in a very primitive way. The tongue perhaps is an expression of hope, a sign from the body ego, that there is some life inside D. D was catatonic, perhaps his body was coming to the rescue. There was no embodiment of D's experience, so it comes out in in these bodily symptoms. Paying attention to the body in treatment of psychotic patient is very important. Proto thoughts or experiences start in the body, like emotions start in body, they can only become feelings when they can be thought about, symbolized, reflected upon and communicated.

Ben Roth while struggling seems intrigued by the case maintaining ongoing interest, and a feeling of suspense as conveyed through the curiosity he has in his patient. He seems attuned to an awareness, that everything in the session is a communication, and it seems this is the seriousness with which Roth attends to his patient to his own thoughts, and to a measure of faith in the "unknown" and unknowable (Bion and Mawson, 2014). Similarly, D is intrigued as he plays games with Roth too.

An external world does not seem to exist for D. Like all psychotic patients, D attacks his own mind and gets rid of awareness of reality. This has resulted in his psychic death. Roth's associations, actions, and mirroring awakens some movement in D's psychotic void, as Roth grapples with this state of no "body," transforming his own thinking for and to himself. He observes or notes the fluctuations within himself, his patient, the hospital staff (e.g., his rise in anxiety, his thought about the unorthodoxy of his manner of speaking to his patient), all of which enable Dr. Roth to feel that he does exist in some way as a "some body." It seems by existing, Roth is holding in mind the nonpsychotic part of D.

Can we presume that there is transference toward the analyst, and if so, it might not necessarily be related to the person of this specific analyst given that the patients contact with reality is deficient. Psychotic patients relate in an undifferentiated way, like D. The analyst is like a sack of projections, not someone with his own personality. Roth notes, "he did not attempt to put meaning together, nor try to understand anything D was saying beyond the surface." Roth simply let himself just exist with his patient, be alive, and as responsive as he could be to what he was listening to and observing.

Roth seemed to register unconsciously at that time, as a young psychotherapist, that a psychotic patient is not capable of a relationship, other than a surface one, as he has no ability to represent his experiences, symbolize them, or reflect upon them. Therefore, he intuited that communication is concrete, and is about the parts of a psychotic patients own mind, not about the relationship to the analyst nor an external object. This one-person relationship, rather than a two person relationship, is however perplexing, as D does seem to have an awareness, perhaps not of the "person of the analyst" but of some aspect of the analyst or an echo of himself in the analyst. D demonstrates this by his responses, and by the fact that he did find language to use once an external reliable frame was in place (ongoing sessions, same psychotherapist, etc.).

D's nonpsychotic mind was able to glimpse the nonpsychotic mind of the analyst, the echo of two sane people talking about what it is like to feel insane. He can't see the person of the analyst because a person is a whole entity, and D can't think in those terms that he is too fragmented, and his functioning is at a part object level.

For the analyst to get close to the psychosis, he has to be receptive to what the patient is doing to him (it's a physical thing), while retaining awareness of his nonpsychotic parts. This is an enormous, difficult task, one that requires time, patience, and skill on the part of the analyst who needs to be able to receive the psychotic projections. The analyst has to do the work on himself or herself, to retain any awareness of the nonpsychotic parts of the patient.

Translating psychotic communications backward to the neurotic origins of the illness is a very difficult but necessary activity (Williams, personal communication). With less disturbed patients, a trauma in early infancy might have been contained while with more psychotic patients when no or little containment has taken place, the neurotic anxiety gets further amplified and escalates into a psychosis, which becomes the quasi resolution to the problem. Psychosis is the ego's last attempt at containment of the crisis using psychotic imagery or psychotic ways of thinking to try and manage what is unmanageable in the absence of a containing object. In other words, the scale of the problem can be on a continuum from less to more severe, from neurotic to psychotic (Williams, P, personal communication).

In the third session, Roth comments "nobody talks to you," and D smiles and says "Gone." This gives the impression that there is a very elementary squiggle game taking place and Roth allows it to remain unsaturated, so as not to bombard his patient with any more than he and his patient can cope with. Why does D smile? Roth is sympathetic when he says "nobody talks to you," indicating via his comment, that he recognizes D is neglected or lonely. Is D's smile a defensive response, that is, his way of saying "nobody can get to me." Paradoxically, it is a horrendous experience to be gone. A part of D does not want to be "gone" as he is in the room talking to Roth and listening to him. I suspect that one can see in that exchange a lot of pain and suffering in D with his inappropriate smile. Perhaps he can't fully smile as it would be too painful. He hears Roth communicate a truth, "nobody talks to you." Does D's own reaction to this truth, become unpalatable and so he smiles at Dr. Roth and says "gone." implying "don't think you can find me." A voice in D says that Roth, talks to him and gives him orders. This I think is the psychotic part of the personality (in loco parentis). These voices act as a quasi-container of anxiety.

Paul William describes a state of "Gone" as a loss of internal life at its core, where the soul has been murdered and is unpopulated and vacant. He suggests this state of oblivion exists prior to psychosis. The person doesn't really exist, Williams suggests, and isn't relating to anybody. Might D be on some continuum between Gone and Psychosis?

The image that appeared in the occupational therapist's room seemed to be a bizarre object (large-beaked bird's head like an eagle on a huge bear like frame, with alligator feet and large lobster claws for hands) – an image of something unsightly and quite absurd. Although heartbreaking to hear of the violent manner in which it was destroyed, its clay quality, hardened and brittle so easily smashed into nothing, brought to my mind upon reading Roth's notes, the psychotic core which, when pierced by human contact, might crash resulting in an emotional breakdown that reveals a fractured internal world.

Another possibility is that D creates an image in the room and has mixed feelings about his creation. The creature is lively and the whole experience of creating something represents being alive, even if the picture is scary. D is attached to the image, but also might feel terrified about destroying it, despite feeling safer doing so. Roth relays how D responds to the trauma of the awful destruction of the image, by becoming catatonic again, regressing, as if he is revisiting a nightmare both in sleep and in his waking life, too disturbing to think or speak about. The catatonia might be how D reverts to a state of deadness as a form of protection, by destroying his creation. It gets projected into the occupational therapist who gets him to smash it. Perhaps the occupational therapist in this sense, carries the destructive and psychotic part of D, at that moment.

Had the occupational therapist had a sense of psychoanalytic process, he might have posed a question such as this to D: *"How would it help you to smash it and how would it feel if you didn't smash it"*. A comment such as this would be a way of trying to engage with the two sides of D so as to prompt him to think about the two side of himself. Instead, D reacts to the projection of panic he might have felt when he created something, to bring himself relief. If a person can dream, mentalize, and give meaning to their omnipotence and destructive phantasies, they do not need to act them out, unlike D who set his house on fire and destroyed his creation. Reality and phantasy blended into one.

Toward the end of the paper, Dr. Roth refers to imagination. Is it possible for a psychotic patient to have an imagination? While all patients can have phantasies, it seems to me that imagination is of a different order, requiring a more developed, less primitive mind, a thought and a thinker, internally not just externally, who can transform the thought creatively, and recognize it as such. D was not able to do that.

The work with D seems to end abruptly due to pressure placed by the hospital on Roth to finish. As a reader I was left wondering about how disruptive this might have been for D. I finished the paper reminded of nobody, nowhere, and gone. D. was discharged by the hospital authorities without consulting Roth about this decision. I wondered where is D now . . . where did he go and what's happened to him? He is a person, but the treatment ended, and if nobody has followed him up, and nobody knows anything about him, what does it say about gone? . . .

Has he gone again?

References

Bion, W. R., and Mawson, C. (2014) *The Complete Works of W. R. Bion.* Routledge. London.

Williams, P. (2013) *Scum.* Routledge. London.

Williams, P. (2021) *The Authority of Tenderness.* Abingdon: Routledge. London

Winnicott, D. W. (2016) *The Collected Works of D. W. Winnicott, Volume 6, 1960–1963.* Oxford University Press. London.

7   Gone

Paul Williams

When you die at a young age, strange things happen. Most are out of reach but the strangest and most paradoxical of them is being unaware that it has happened while at the same time experiencing it each moment. This could be thought of as 'Gone'. Not Gone temporarily or in search of an alternative but Gone never to return. There may be different ways Gone can come about, like infant suicide or the crushing of a soul, but whatever form it takes, two things need to occur at the same time. One is being unoccupied or uninhabited. There is no one, inside or out, to see what is taking place. The second is an experience of inner violence so intense as to give rise to a paralyzing of imagination. I am uninhabited, I am inundated. This is not the same as psychosis, though this may ensue. Gone exists prior to psychosis and denotes a loss of life at its core. GONE Absence of interest in the Gone child concentrates subjective experience in bodily action. Nothing is what it seems, a lack of comprehension so sweeping that objects are reified as either inscrutable or threatening. A tree is harmless until it rains, a bus a dog-fight pit, car an intergalactic missile, body a machine, shit a shocking punishment, food a conspiracy, sky sheet metal, and so on. Misrecognition on this scale prevents learning, a deficit felt bodily, the body of an automaton, not a deficit taken in mentally, because the learning process has not been learned. I know what I already knew – physical pandemonium. The world of Gone is raw, outside space and time, consisting of upheaval frozen in the nothing it represents. Indifference, the precursor to Gone, is a vacuum force unlike anything else. From nowhere, indifference activates a gravitational vortex that whips craving into a planetary cyclone, like Jupiter's Great Red Spot.[1] Predicated on the actuality of nothing, indifference views as axiomatic the destruction of everything that is not itself. Without prescience of something that anything else might be the scheme could miscarry, so an equation everything – not everything – nothing dismantles the problem of everything and its loss at its inception, in the needs of an infant. The effect of indifference might seem akin to neglect, but neglect fails in its lethargic unconcern to convey the resolve needed to achieve indifference. Annihilation of need requires doggedness and ingenuity. 42 GONE The outcome, for both parties, is barrenness scarred by vestiges of butchery, a landscape beyond neglect.

DOI: 10.4324/9781003427049-8

Indifference renders me the last remaining life form of a desecrated land. The Gone child, unable to know anything, cannot learn or change. Some may learn something from experience, but if the learning apparatus is stillborn, adaptation is the sole option, there being no one available to learn anything. From the basic facts of life – birth, development, and death – to the stuff of life between is a closed book to the Gone child who adopts the least harrowing stance – indifference. A swell of grievance or pining indicating hope that Gone need not be forever propels Gone's chilling tide of apathy to drown what remains. Indifference is not the prerogative of the ill. Parents, schoolteachers, public servants, clerics, young people – all of us can display indifference if truth proves to be indigestible. This encourages further concealment by the Gone child. Consider the discernment and prudence needed to identify, let alone engage with, Gone. Everything has Gone. The residual nothingness before you that passes for a life form could stand for anything, from shy or withdrawn to woebegone, depraved or insane, depending upon its ramshackle presentation. Who cares anyway? The Gone child walks, turns up, leaves, goes 'home', day after day, week after week, doesn't it? What is there to say? 43 GONE A Gone child makes imperceptible yet overwhelming demands, is unmanageable and is disappeared. Insensibility is their first order of business. Any communication is on the lines of: 'Gone. Desperate. Return under no circumstances. Stop'. Rules of engagement of a rational kind run aground immediately. The only thing, the dreadful thing, that offers a hope of correspondence lies in our willingness to experience what it is like to feel Gone. The Gone condition, founded upon absolute mistrust, takes nothing for granted: no analyst, authority, talk, gesture. It fumbles helplessly for some unidentified, putative ally who will suspend belief, tolerate disarray, suffer incongruous, unjustified assaults, breathe a toxic, confounding fog and be willing to suffer an experience of ruination. Small wonder Gone people are inconspicuous and loath to elicit concern. Smaller wonder still they deter the mental health profession. The Gone individual anticipates ostracism and neither you nor I grasp the sheer number of ways in which this is inflicted. We have to be taught. Whatever shape the induction takes, it is a rite de passage not to be confused with torture, despite the resemblances. The injunction is that we be taken out of ourselves in a way not previously experienced and traverse the path of Gone at as many intersection points as we can bear. Mercifully, the Gone individual cannot tolerate exposure for long, so the process is paced and cyclical. 44 GONE I/she/he need infinite space and time to formulate a second communication: 'Gone. Desperate. Return under no circumstances. Stop. Go'. I dread my susceptibility to this hubris, kindling of spent ashes, but I ask you for help anyway, an unthinkable idea, and you accede. Delusional. Dismay at your many presumptions plunges me into insentience. You are insane. Is anything real? Am I alive? Dead? Dead while breathing? In trying to negotiate in bare feet ice pinnacles and gales, crossroads, and so-called meeting points, I throw a sidelong glance in acknowledgment, in the certainty that you will die, suddenly or little by little, as you mistakenly accept, and fail to mistakenly accept, desecration that befouls and pauperizes. For me, torture, stabbing, terror. For you, vexation, degeneracy, impotence. The doomed folly cannot go on. Goes on. I kill, you suffer, I kill. To what end? Perhaps a difference between this lunacy and Gone might be I am not Gone. Meeting points, of which I have no knowledge, contravene Gone. I do not seek friendship or understanding. These ideas appall me. I do not know who you are, who anyone is. I don't want to know. Or to not know. I don't want. I need you to accept only that I am Gone. I don't know I need this, so I don't know you know or don't know I need this and don't know. 45 GONE No guidance, instruction, help. Just pinnacles, gales, crossing points, menace. I fear, hate, cower, abscond but do not know I misread. I do not know that you know or do not know that I misread and do not know. Filth, stigma, misery. The light drip of acceptance unfelt. Your frustration, resentment, boredom, indifference are proof you do not, cannot, care. You cannot suffer such calumny: no one can, other than me. What is the point? Tantalizing inferences at crossroads you will recite for years unless I put a stop to it. At one intersection a mighty collision triggers a multiple pileup. Smoke, flames, burning wrecks. I run for my life but before I can get away I am questioned by police and paramedics about what happened. Outraged, I fucking tell them what happened. No charges are pressed. I am lucky to be alive. Thanks a lot. You? A drawn-out inquest investigates the death of a child, a serious matter, so every detail has to be Gone through. Meanwhile, more crossing points, near misses, no smashes, for now. Why on earth risk it again? I appear to have had to change direction, or driving style, or something as I see the problem lies not just with my annihilation but in making you see that you are, I now know, out of your mind. And so on. 46 GONE At intersections divergent realities collide, never in exactly the same way, instigating a thousand different outcomes, loud, soft, dark, bright, great, small, imperceptible. I see some but not others. My body returns unbidden. Points of intersection, terrifying, shameful, enraging, accrue, yet beckon my body and me (?) to accept you (?) are there, I (?) am there and accept you (?) accept I (?) am there. This is unwelcome. To think you (?) know me (?), accept me (?), incenses me. I can negotiate crossroads. I can appear to listen. I know what works. Work. In Gone there is only work, work to stave off death. What worked works. My body may turn up, but I work. I am sickened that shame and fear dominate my life, whatever that is. Let me put this candidly. I have no interest in what you say. A holding pattern is needed to put what I know to better use. Realism. The holding pattern, too close to Gone, does not silence dreams of being lost and abominated. You notice with your usual contrivances, feeble surmises, my body insolently returns. I do not accept this. Must I endure more nothing when I know nothing works? Did I not accept this? 47 GONE Why did you accept this when you had a job to do? I am to accept this? Accept me? Accept you? Accept nothing I accept? Dreams. Defeat, appalling decisions, a thousand forfeited opportunities, longings, grief. The themes repeat themselves, crisscrossing each other. Did you know this? I no longer see which theme is which, not that I ever could. Did you? Crisscrossing?

Crossing Points? Crossroads? Am I missing something? I talked about this, didn't I? I'm sure I did. Did you hear? You replied. Was this me (?) speaking, you (?) listening? You (?) speaking, me (?) listening? What were the thousand intersections? A thousand lost opportunities? A thousand lethal injections? Neither? Were you (?) there? You (?) accepted them? Accepted me (?)? You (?) present? 48 GONE Me (?) present? You (?) accept me (?) Gone?

Note

1 A spinning, anticyclonic storm twice the size of Earth, believed to have existed for at least 350 years, producing wind speeds of 425 mph and temperatures of 2420°F. Different, freezing variations surround Saturn with winds of 1,500 mph and temperatures of −280°F.

8 Working in the dark and from the heart

Anthony Bass

Young Bennett E. Roth's encounter with D, as Dr. Roth recalls some 50 years later, was an unusual and formative event in his becoming the psychotherapist and psychoanalyst that he is today. The seeds of that future creative psycho-analyst, just beginning to sprout when he met that troubled boy were evident from the start: "While I was untrained in formal psychotherapy, in retrospect I appeared to have respected the boundaries of his vulnerable self." "Respect for the boundaries of a vulnerable self" is a sine qua non of working non-traumatically with our most vulnerable patients, a quality that guided Roth's work from the start. His supervisors at the inpatient facility in which he saw D for that brief time that made such an impression on Ben (and I imagine on D too) saw his natural, yet to be trained talent and supported Roth in his efforts to reach this silent boy in unconventional, risky, and experimental ways.

Roth was "flying by the seat of his pants," with honesty, working with his young patient from his heart, and in the dark. He asks, "what role did my honest ignorance play in his treatment" of D? The unselfconscious honest ignorance of a beginning therapist combined with his authentic wish to make a difference in a troubled person's life may be the secret sauce in the good work that young therapists so often do with their patients. For those who have been in practice for many years, it is often harder to come by, but coming to terms with how little we know about another person remains an important source of therapeutic humility and openness that stands us in good stead throughout our lifetimes. In coming to terms with the limits of what we know, about another person who is our patient and about parts of ourselves that are activated in our encounter with our patient remain an important source of our curiosity and openness to new experience and learning, and our capacity to meet each patient where they are, and to accept that our patient meets us where we are too.

Many of us look back on our earliest encounters with patients, when we had little or no training, as the most difficult, challenging, mind opening, fright-ening, and enlightening experiences of our professional lives. Such experi-ences remain with us throughout our lives, occupy our reveries and dreams, and inform us as we work with our patients and supervisees over the decades. I think of my first patients often, wondering how their lives have gone – did

DOI: 10.4324/9781003427049-9

our encounter makes a difference. It did for me. Yalom's novel "The Schopenhauer Cure" begins with the narrator receiving a fatal medical diagnosis, and finding that part of his preparation for death, and considering what his life has amounted to, decides to get in touch with the most difficult patients he has treated, those with whom he had struggled the most, to find out how they "had done" in life, what had become of them. In the process, his own life was enriched as he achieved greater self-awareness as his life came to an end.

What became of Ben's D, I wonder. Did his experience of finding someone worth talking to, coming out of silence for in his therapist, however brief the time they had together, lead to more access to his thoughts and others' that set his life on a path in which other ways of expressing himself and relating to others would become possible? Dr. Roth's recollections of his encounter with D evoked several of my own earliest encounters with patients whom I did my best to help and to find before I had any professional training – I think about these patients now, almost 50 years later, I hold them in mind, wondering how their life unfolded. Occasionally a patient has found me after many years away, most recently one who returned after a 30-year hiatus. The man whom he had become wanted to pick up where the boy that he had been with me left off. In our second chance at therapy, we have each been learning more about who we were then and who we are now. I wish there had been a second chapter to Ben and D's story, that they could have met up for more work and that they each could have taken their conversation further than their first brief encounter had allowed. Could D have told Ben more about what had happened to him that brought him to their first encounter, as my patient filled me in on what he could not tell me has a young college student? Ralph Linder, a favorite supervisor of mine during my internship years at the VA hospital in Brooklyn, where I saw many of my first, most disturbed patients, used to say to his young trainees,

> as you are seeing your patients here, try to forget all that smart stuff you have been learning in graduate school. All this freshly learned theory – I know you are all very good at it – will get in your way, as much as it will help you. You will probably help them more if you forget it while you are with them, and be the way your favorite grandparent was with you, caring and interested in you.

As Dr. Roth points out, had he been in the thick of training and reading and learning theory as he would soon be, at the time he encountered D, it might have interfered with the very way of being with him that seemed to have played an important part in D's beginning to come out of his silence. As he said:

> in analytic training it seemed that there was a distance from the patient and that the pathology was explained at some distance in the patient's past. I felt more comfortable working in close to what the patient expressed in the room.

Roth was in uncharted territory, spontaneous, puzzled, and experimental. As he noted, "I don't think I would have been able to explain what I did other than to admit that I did not want him to be alone and in danger?" That is not a bad way to begin any therapeutic relationship, even if being alone together at some point becomes possible when there is enough of a self to tolerate it without dissociating from the experience. It is indeed dangerous to be alone when there is not a good enough internal object to supply safe accompaniment. I think, Roth sensed that this was the case with D even without having the object relations theory to back him up, but he was informed by what he intuitively understood.

D's occupational therapist reported that D was under psychic threat, but didn't elaborate the nature of the threat other than to say "his eyes were under attack." I imagined that the "eyes" under attack may have stood as well for his (I's) those first personal singular subjective case (Is), or selves, as fragmented as they might have been, under attack from both outside and in. Roth noted that calling out "nobody" to appear, not to hide, was a challenging way of demonstrating to D that he wasn't on "the outside" and in particular "that he was not real to me." As an interpersonal relational analyst, I take it for granted that no two therapists would have the same patient, and that no two patients would have the same therapist. Ben's D would not be another therapists D, and my D would not be Ben's. Each therapy couple, at whatever stage of the work, and no matter how brief, constitutes some coming together of the two psyches at work and play in the field of therapy.

As I used my own imagination to find my way to my own D (imagining my young self with this young patient), I believe I would be cautious in calling out "nobody" to appear and not to hide, because I would consider whether he might feel that his life depended on the cover that his "nobody" persona provided. Was D a wily Greek hero Ulysses, a master of disguise, who when he encountered the ravenous and deadly Greek eating Cyclops Polyphemus, cleverly disguised his identify under the moniker "Nobody." Ulysses and his men then plied Polyphemus with wine until he fell into a deep sleep, and then attacked **his** eyes with a fire hardened shaft that took out his one eye, leaving him blind. Polyphemus groped in the dark for his tormentors, but the Greeks dodged him all night long. When morning came, he called out for help "I am blinded and in agony." "Whose fault is this," they responded. "Nobody's, Polyphemus shouted back." "Well, why are you bothering us," they shouted, as Ulysses and his men escaped with their lives. Was D the Cyclops whose eyes could be pierced by the trickster, or the trickster who could be somebody, a hero in fact, but Nobody when necessary to save his own skin. As both "Nobody" and the Cyclops whose eyes (I's) were under attack, D may have been both hero and monster, perpetrator and victim, somebody when it was safe and nobody when it was safer, with his therapist invited to assume the complementary roles in turn. As Ben played the lovable champ Ali, unafraid but with a bit of playful self-deprecation as he played a "poor imitation" of the champ himself,

D responded with a smile. Perhaps he recognized himself in B's funny act, a champ playing the fool and a fool playing a champ. Like D, Ben could play a slightly less graceful Ali, or a Cowardly Lion, or a Cyclops or Ulysses, just as D could play the one-eyed monster whose eye could be pierced by Ulysses, or the trickster who escapes under the cover of being Nobody.

Ben imagined that their finding a way to be together without mayhem or murder was the turning point to D's getting better. "Maybe that will be able to help him." As I imagine the scene, I think that the question of who is protecting whom from what murder or mayhem by what part of one or the other of us remains something of an open question, potentially to be determined as we come more able to put our thoughts and feelings into words, if we were fortunate enough to have the time and mental space to manage that. Ben's feeling that D was fooling him may have carried a countertransference suggestion that D was Ben's Ulysses, Ben the Cyclops who could blind D if he could only find him. If that is the case, being found is a double-edged sword for them both, as either B or D could commit mayhem or be blinded in the finding or being found. As Winnicott put it, "it is a joy to be hidden, and disaster not to be found" (1965). With a boy like D, it might be a disaster to be found, and a disaster to stay hidden. As Winnicott might also say, these disasters that are enacted in the brief therapy encounter between D and Ben may be reflective of disasters that have already occurred in the young man's life, but have not yet been fully experienced (1974). Their reenactment is a way of keeping them present until he finds a safe enough place to encounter the disaster in consciousness. If this is the case, a full therapy would be what he would need to have one day to foster his potential to come back to life.

How important is the question of diagnosis in cases such as this? I am not sure. Diagnosis is an important frame of reference in thinking about what medication might be helpful. But in reaching another person, in finding a way to understand and to be understood by him, a diagnosis might constitute one of those ways of finding distance from another person that Ben was rightfully wary of. Ben seemed to have acquired to diagnosis of catatonia having catatonia, because he didn't speak. As I imagined D's toy soldier walk, and the way he walked in place after hitting the barrier of the closed door, I imagined a boy on the autistic spectrum, a bit of an automaton, programed to walk more like a toy soldier, or robot boy who continues to walk in place when he hit the barrier of a closed door, than a real boy who knows intuitively to stop in front of a closed door. Either way, catatonia or autism spectrum disorder, Ben's job was to find him "where he lived," the diagnostic manual providing a less clear signal than his own heart.

Weeks passed in heir being alone together, each in their own separate world, before the significant communication took place, of D rolling his tongue out like a lizard. Ben approximated the movement as best he could. It was as though Ben were encountering a kind of Extra Terrestrial, and saying, "Welcome, I am here and will try to speak your language."

That exchange of physical mirroring or mimicry seemed to be the portal into the next phase of the therapy work.

Rot said, "Who told you to do that?"
He said, "Nobody told me."
I said, "No body told me"
He said, "You speak to nobody?"
I said "You speak to nobody?"
He said, "Nobody speaks to me"
I said, "No body speaks to me"
He said, "Nobody tells me what to do"
I said, "No body tells me what to do or say"
He laughed and said, "Nobody tells me what to say." (page 6)

Their exchange, that even included a laugh of apparent recognition (remarkable in either a catatonic or autistic boy), seemed like the beginning of a quite important communication. If they had the time, it might have even been, as Rick said to Louie in the last scene of Casablanca, "Louie, I think this is the beginning of a beautiful friendship." Or, the beginning of a deepening therapy relationship.

Their exchange of repetitions and the slight and quite subtle variations that evoked a laugh in D brought to my mind Sanford Meisner's repetition exercise (aka the word repetition game) which requires an actor to sit across from their scene partner and make an observation about them. The scene partner then repeats the observation back. This exercise aims to create a connection between the actors by ensuring that they are actively listening to one another. Meisner described it as a ping-pong game that becomes the foundation for emotional connection.

Initially, the actors begin by repeating the exact same sentence, such as "You're looking at me." Then, they advance to repeating the observation from their own points of view, as in "You're looking at me," followed by the other actor saying, "I'm looking at you." Or, if the actor is not looking at their scene partner, they could respond, "I'm not looking at you." The Meisner repetition exercise then grows into an entire scene of naturalistic, improvised dialogue.

Such scenes between Ben and D seem to me to constitute their own discovery of a kind of emotional preparation and way of connecting that have the potential to set an autistic or catatonic or psychotic boy on a path to beginning to connect, even in an inchoate way, with another person, as Ben and D were beginning to do in the above-cited passage.

Here is another exchange that moves their emotional connection further along:

"Where is No body" I began.
"He is gone".
"Where is No body?"
"He is gone"

"Where is gone?"

"I am gone"

"You are Gone:"

"You are Gone?" I repeat.

He replied, "I am gone now".

"You are gone now."

"I was Blind," he continued.

I was surprised by the term and hesitated.

"Blind?"

"I was blind".

"Blind." You can't see?".

"Show yourself don't be no where."

They plunge further into what is beginning to look a lot like play:

"I stand up and I do an imitation of Burt Lahr as the Cowardly Lion." Oh Yea come on out and I will fight you. I ain't afraid of you. I ain't afraid of no body. No body come on and fight me. Come on out. Don't hide you coward I will fight you with one hand behind my back (I am standing now and assume a boxers stance) Come on out you nobody. You are afraid nobody. Show yourself. Don't hide; I will fight you with two hands behind my back." Shuffling into boxer stance. "You're the one afraid," and then I do an Ali shuffle. "Come on out you mangy coward and fight me. Sting like a Bee, float like a butterfly. I am the greatest."

D looks unafraid, smiles, and says: "Nobody will get you."

They were beginning to play, even somewhat aggressively, and it was beginning to make a difference. D started attending school, and sat with other boys at lunch, even if awkwardly.

Ben took risks to be with D on his own terms, even risking the censure of his employers by joining D in a pee over the dead bird. Ben mirrored D in ways that calmed D down, stopped his shaking. He took a "different rout" to protect D from the terror of encountering death.

The bidirectionality of Ben's force as protector from both reality and internal attacker was revealed in their co-constructed choreography and incantations around the dead bird. He had to be light on his feet to manage this, like Ali himself, floating like a butterfly, stinging like a bee, as needed. Ben managed in his shadow play to show how the greatest, the champ, Mohammed Ali himself, slayer of dragons (Liston) and Cyclops, was really not so different from the Cowardly Lion, a dreamed – up figure who could play both the fighter and the fool. D's revelation that he was, among other things, blind, evoked the image of another mythological figure, John Lennon's No Where man. Not only were D and B, in part Nobodies, in addition to be Somebodies, but they were also Nowhere Men, even as they were each on their way to finding their place "somewhere." And as John Lennon wrote, that man is not only Ben and D, but also you and me.

D's No One, his No Where man has found, fortunately for him, someone to lend him a hand, in Ben. He does not yet know where he is going, has not developed a sense of his own subjectivity sufficiently to have a point of view he can call his own (or the voices in his head carry perhaps multiple points of view at war with each other). Ben wonders if D can see him at all, and I would wonder too, who is the blind man among us. Therapy is often a matter of the blind leading the blind, where recognizing one's blindness is part of beginning to see for therapist and patient alike. Ben is seeing if he can lead D out of the darkness to discover that he is inhabited by more than No Body, and that he is not only "nowhere." D is leading Ben through the maze of his earliest experiences treating deeply troubled people as human beings worth finding a way to talk to and to help to find a path that will play no small part in his becoming the seasoned therapist he would become. For therapist and patient alike, it felt at times that D and the voices and differing self-states that he carried with him were beyond reach. One thing they didn't have enough of was time to complete what might under other circumstances have been a bigger mission toward a fuller life, and so John Lennon's injunction not to worry and to take their time doesn't quite fit the picture that began to develop between Ben and D. I would like to imagine that D would find B again one day and catch him up on all that has transpired, since they went their separate ways.

References

Winnicott, D. W. (1965) Communicating and Not Communicating Leading to a Study of Certain Opposites (1963). PP 179–192 *The Maturational Processes and the Facilitating. EnvironMENT* The International Psychoanalytic Library, London.

Winnicott, D. W. (1974) Fear of Breakdown. *International Review of Psychoanalysis* 1:103–107.

9 On trust as a necessary precondition to therapeutic success

Priscilla F. Kauff

I did not think I could explain what started him talking.

Dr. Ben Roth

The question has been asked as to how verbal communication was achieved with a 15-year-old adolescent catatonic boy who had not spoken in two years. There is no single answer to such an inquiry of course. Furthermore, the question raises a complex, insufficiently explored topic, namely the mysterious nature of successful connections between therapist and patient.

The comments below will, almost entirely, be related to Dr. Roth's own reports of his experience, internally and behaviorally, as to his interaction with the patient. I will not attempt to unpack the psychodynamics of the interaction which is addressed elsewhere. The focus of this discussion will be upon the development of *trust* between Dr. Roth and patient D. Identifying the observable elements in the ultimately successful connection between them should at least begin to shed some light upon this important topic.

In general, people of all ages are likely to experience a stranger in a strange situation with a fair amount of uncertainty if not *mistrust*. Indeed, it might be argued that such an attitude is appropriate at least initially. The necessity of overcoming such lack of trust poses one of the most difficult challenges to the initiation (and ultimately to the success of) every therapeutic relationship.

Despite his avowed lack of training and experience at the time, Dr. Roth was able to develop a condition of trust which in turn enabled patient D to overcome the severe constrictions of his illness and begin to engage in verbal interaction. While it is impossible to specify every element of this process, a close look at what Dr. Roth has reported may help to clarify at least some of the basic ingredients.

"Trust" is defined here as the belief that you are not in danger of being harmed, either by the circumstances in which you find yourself or by the person(s) involved. Trust is generally experienced as a feeling of comfort, with a minimum of anxiety as to ones' physical and psychological well-being. The development of this condition in the therapy situation can take a very short

DOI: 10.4324/9781003427049-10

time, but it may extend to the end of treatment and perhaps beyond. Trust may also expand into a belief that circumstances/people can make things *better* than they are at the start – that is, not simply result in the avoidance of a bad outcome.

Since trust in the therapeutic situation exists between at least two people, the capacity of each of them to engage in its development is critical. Both the degree to which a patient is actually receptive to the therapist's efforts as well as the therapist's professional skill are required. Not surprisingly, there are many occasions in which the players themselves preclude the development of trust from the start. Fortunately, in this case, D was catatonic but not catastrophically resistant and Dr. Roth seems to have instinctively brought the right ingredients to the recipe.

Dr. Roth's detailed description of his interaction with D allows us to speculate as to what he did and did not do that was so effective in initiating the trust required to make a positive connection. Fortunately, it was apparent from the start that there was at least a minimal permeability in D's catatonia, as indicated by his response to Dr. Roth calling out his name. He stood up . . . "with a fixed smile on his face . . . walked like a toy soldier . . . walked in place in front of the closed door . . . and . . . stood the entire time." The mere response to his name, robotic though it may have looked, may have been the first indication of the patient's receptivity to possible future connection. Though it appeared mechanical and indeed painful, there was a great deal of nonverbal interaction in this initial contact that was allowed to unfold at the patient's pace, *without* a negative response of any kind from Dr. Roth. His silent acceptance of the pace and the nature of D's behavior may have spoken volumes to this boy. The "bridge" that Dr. Roth believed necessary to make contact with D, which he describes as "safe attention and a resonating environment," began at this point.

Over a period of about three weeks, positive aspects of the therapist's presence and behavior resulted in the productive interchange that began with D's sticking his tongue out at Dr. Roth, who returned the gesture. I believe Dr. Roth's imitation of the patient's behavior was a further assurance of safety. He welcomed the patient's communication as understandable and acceptable. This occurred after Dr. Roth described having sat with D "doing and saying nothing." It can certainly be speculated that "nothing" was more likely "something" in this case! Dr. Roth's capacity to refrain from acting on his own agenda, his ability to do "nothing," is a testament to what I believe is a necessary precondition for a positive therapeutic condition. Speculative dynamic hypothesizing and planned treatment interventions would have directly interfered with Dr. Roth's ultimately successful approach.

While the dynamics of the extraordinary interchange between Dr. Roth and D around "Nobody" deserve the attention that it will surely get from other contributors, I think that it was in part a consequence of the trust that had already developed between them. It was *also* a confirmation of the trust that D was feeling and no doubt served to deepen it as well. Dr. Roth exercised extremely careful attention to the patient's peculiar use of words. It required strenuous effort to understand the idiosyncratic ways in which the patient's words could reflect his disturbed internal life. That Dr. Roth cared enough to make that effort was consistently obvious and undoubtedly a contributing factor to the developing trust.

The first overt gesture initiated by Dr. R to D was his offer of a piece of chewing gum which seemed to be ignored It is fair to speculate that D registered the gesture, responding physically but not verbally, perhaps waiting to see what would come next. What came next was that Dr. Roth continued to wait for D to venture out, without a demand related either to the chewing gum or to anything else. In turn, D made no demands upon Dr. Roth. Clearly Dr. Roth was paying very close attention to D's nonverbal signals and responding to them creatively in such a way did not threaten the patient. Furthermore, it seems reasonable to assume that offering him the gum was a concrete act of caring/feeding without any expectation of return, and with nothing negative to follow. This was all in the context of Dr. Roth deliberately refraining from touching the patient – which again is a strong nonverbal assurance of physical safety at the least.

The verbal contact began with the memorable "no body . . . nobody" sequences. It should be noted that three weeks had passed. There is no question that time matters . . . some amount of time is required for the parties to suspend judgment or at least to resolve interpersonal anxiety enough to begin to trust one another. In this case, it is clear that any catastrophic expectations D may have harbored were *never* met with catastrophic responses from Dr. Roth. Repeated over time, this interaction was surely fundamental to the trust that developed.

As analysts, we rarely look at our physical selves to appraise how we may appear to a patient except when challenged by our patients' observations or transference enactments. Another possible factor in the development of trust with D is Dr. Roth's physical presence. Dr. Roth's size and usually calm demeanor may have been a factor in the patient's willingness to trust him once he became assured that the powerful figure in the room was not going to turn this "strength" against him. The patient seemed to reflect this when he called Dr. Roth "Ben Equally Strong." I believe it is clear that the patient experienced Dr. Roth as sufficient to the task of protecting either one or both of them from whatever threat was present or may have arisen in the future.

Dr. Roth makes references to the notion that . . . A listening other is the requirement for strands of trust to form a bridge between the participants so that safe emotional exchanges can take place. He also paraphrases Marcus (2017) by stating that certain patients "need a witness, a friend, a bystander or human sponge for their anxiety or violent thoughts." Fortunately, Dr. Roth served these functions instinctively when, at this early phase in his career, he was confronted with such a severely disturbed patient. The ability to do so is a talent, which if absent in a therapist can be taught to some and not to others.

In conclusion, trust that is established and maintained over the course of treatment is considered to be an absolute requirement for the successful progress of treatment. There is no bucket list of characteristics pertaining to the therapist, the patient or specifics of the therapeutic situation that will guarantee the development of trust. However, at least two factors emerge in this case as particularly significant:

1   the therapist's ability to maintain a neutral, accepting, and nondemanding presence, giving priority to the patient's agenda and timing over his own;
2   the patient's freedom to express his thoughts and feelings, negative though they may be in his estimation, without suffering real or imagined catastrophic consequences.

These factors taken together are fundamental, indeed irreducible. Understandably, a period of time (that will vary from case to case) is required for the process to evolve. In addition, the availability of both parties, that is, the receptivity of the patient and the effective participation of the therapist are necessary. Finally, the therapist's ability to pay unqualified, accepting attention to the unique form and content of the patient's communications must dictate the actual details of the therapeutic interaction. When successful – as in the present case – the possibility that patients like D will be enabled to "start talking" – to commence direct communication – is greatly enhanced.

Reference

Marcus E, R (2017) Psychosis and Near Psychosis: Ego Function, Symbol Structure, Treatment Routledge. London.

Discussion

Bennett E. Roth

The reconstruction of my early psychotherapy encounter with a catatonic boy was a learning experience. It is published with the hope of continued learning while generously followed by reflective comments by seasoned therapists of that effort. A dialogue constructed as an "interview with that therapist" also follows it. Where modern psychiatry has resorted to medication with such patients the rich and varied responses to the original case are an attempt to capture the early revolutionary spirit of psychoanalysis with the depiction of a unique "psychoanalytic treatment" in this book.

The reconstructed case was prompted by the appearance of a challenge when I revealed I had treated a catatonic boy in psychotherapy. There is an absence of clinical material of the psychotherapeutic treatment of those suffering or resorting to catatonic behaviors and others like them that exists with the recent stagnation in our field. The required confidentiality of psychotherapy as a unique encounter has the side effect of shielding the highly individual nature of our work while preventing learning from directly observing each other's efforts. The clinical appearance of catatonia often reveals only the surface tip of its iceberg obscuring many windows of therapeutic entrance. The greater unseen structures or dynamics are beneath the manifest sight line are revealed here by the varied possibilities of these viable approaches. The aim of this endeavor is to add to our knowledge of a mystifying unseen illness and rediscover the creative multiplicity of psychoanalytic knowledge. D's mental life may now best be described as engaged in pseudo hallucinations that created an imaginary and alternative reality that demanded his attention. What distinguishes pseudohallucinations from perceptions and hallucinations is that pseudohallucinations appear to "the inner eye" as "pictorial/figurative," that is, with a "character of subjectivity" in the "inner subjective space," in a manner similar to and may replace normal orienting to reality or external voices. D's idiosyncratic imagery appeared as his absorbing obsession while occupying his attention and guiding or directing his behavior away from contacting others in reality with the appearance of being under siege. The creation of an alternative inner reality is likely a result and the process described by Williams (2000).

DOI: 10.4324/9781003427049-11

Paranoia is assumed to rest on projection and projective identification of "parts" of objects and overwhelming identification with rejecting others along with a fear of integration. In D's situation, the usual paranoid fixation from the outside coexisted with internal threats to his existence. He believed, it appeared to me, that he was not safe in reality with others at the same time he was a target of his own thoughts (forces) as described by Paul Williams. Cojoined with the threats D created an internal malignant geographic reality by projection/introjection that was porous in which were threats and hiding places. His was a psychotic world, different in its rules and language from the external world, one in which negation and threat have captured and inverted his thinking. Safety seemed also to be present in his world although being a temporary hiatus from threats.

The ongoing verbal and nonverbal encounters between D and myself were the essential basis for my simple understanding his disorder. Psychotherapy essentially depends on the dynamics of spoken language and the struggle to have safe verbal exchanges in which surface meaning and a unique form of reparative intimacy could be found. While there were a variety of nonverbal communications that took place and likely contributed to the therapeutic trust and contact, spoken language was primarily the source of information and confusion. Consensual references were frequently absent and one striking aspect of this encounter was the therapist's struggle to establish shared meaning enabling communication. It is assumed when treating psychosis in patients that meaningful verbal exchanges of information with shared meaning are problematic. In order to communicate with D I had to learn and use his verbal referents that were infiltrated by either his powerful destructive negative or an oppositional meaning; seemingly originating in a unique internal "object" for him likely formed by or making use of an inner hatred. His alternative reality functioned with alternative meanings with an inverted language.

This change in his reference or to private oppositional language is different from the distortions found in schizophrenic's use of language. Dr. Reiner addresses how the early acquisition of shared language is preempted by the psychic negative from the perspective of Grotstein's (2007) careful clarification of Bion's theory. Bion's theory extended Klein's notion of the early failure of maternal containment and hence disruption of normal projection plays a significant role. She emphasizes that much of what happened in the sessions with D had the quality of being a shared dream as a form of connection despite his self being fragmented. I spoke to him as if he existed in a shared reality. While I had no information of the occasion of D's withdrawal into his private world Karen Todes suggests his setting fire to his home is the likely significant external manifestation of his violent mental upheaval. Her comments also reveal the powerful impact D's psychotic projections likely had on my thinking from the very start of our work together and my mental struggle to stay in verbal contact with him.

Eric R. Marcus emphasizes the therapists' ability to remain a witness to the psychotic upheaval the patient suffers and the process to become a part of the patients' world in which he is frequently targeted. Interestingly he suggests that the therapist seeks to become a transitional object for the patient. In this manner he refines the meaning of my sticking my tongue out as play and playing Burt Lahr in a session as establishing an imaginary object-with words that is in a relationship with D in reality. Such acts offered a "potential space" in which the perception of me and not me can become distinct from his delusions.

Williams carefully illuminates the role of therapist/ witness in the treatment of D, as there were none of the usual significant interpretative interventions usually recognized in psychoanalytic treatment. Perhaps to D I was always a part of an object. Yet this was not a fault in the therapy but the real occasion of essential human contact and willingness to be with D when he was suffering and felt in threatened.

In the usual psychoanalytic atmosphere of more intact patients, not vulnerable to psychosis or soul murder, the therapeutic role of being with a person describing their suffering is often ignored as being necessary. What moved me to silently to "dance around the dead bird with D" was to continue to make eye contact and not abandon him in his unknown unseen crises. Physically communicating, "I am here. With you." Paul Williams understands such crises in the catatonic experience as the recurring product of an internal psychotic process in which the fear of annihilation is lived through an invasive internal object.

Dr. Marcus approached this material from the perspective of Winnicott's deceptively complex ideas of the interacting mother- child unit and reveals the multiplicity of that role in psychotherapy. There is no therapy without a pair: therapist and patient. The therapeutic encounter then becomes a "potential space" for the patient. Perhaps without realizing it Dr. Marcus lends support to the idea of the infant or child who is denied or unable to use an accessible container mother as an anchor in reality into whom to project is more likely to develop a preemptive attacking mental object. In D's mind his "no body" voice offered sadistic security while posing at least an equal destructive threat.

In retrospect one of the major forces that might explain D's recovery was my being uninfluenced by his destructive and threatening projections. D likely had a compulsive need to expel his unbearable violent states of mind embedded in his psychotic state using me as a repository. If I consider his tongue thrusting at the dead bird as being an essential part of a projective evacuative sequence with a malignant origin our relationship started with similar behavior. His violence included the imagined threats to my life that he experienced as dangerous that were absorbed by me. I continued being with him in therapy and he did not to drive me away'

My early inference was that nobody or No-body was a voice without a body in his mind. It emerged as his verbal representation of a destructive force that opposed my presence in D's life. Dr. Bass has much to say about the obscured meaning of No Body in our culture. The lyrics "Your nobody till somebody loves you" ties the notion of the emergence of identity to early love being generative. Bass also juxtaposes the healthy openness, curiosity, and risk-taking of the new therapist with the attitudes that develop with training.

Priscilla F. Kauff emphasizes the nonverbal elements of "being with" as being the elements of trust essential to therapy that often are unrecognized. Her position emphasizes the here and now presence of therapy and being able to absorb D's "threat" in the sessions as earning his essential trust. What matters most in treating such patients' threat is the ability to be emotionally honest with them in the hope of providing a psychological atmosphere of trust, constancy, and acceptance. I believe that trust likely started with sharing his catatonic silence and then treating him as existing in reality with me.

One of the uncanny events in putting this book together was the discovery of William's earlier chapter "Gone." This powerful essay reveals Williams's gift for capturing the agony of being Gone in words. It is a microscope enlarging D's being gone; and the word he used for himself: being made into a no body or of having no body as suggested by Reiner. It was difficult to read the description of not being and the terror to be.

The array of responses to my encounter with D is exquisite and beyond any expectations. I was absorbed for weeks by the material revealed. Uncertainty reigned while elements of the original encounter gave up their possible dynamics. The case became a giant analytic jigsaw puzzle without a boundary pushing at the edges of catatonia, expanding. I waited, knowing that I had an obligation to respond. Then I realized there was an organizing principle: the selected fact. Selected fact is Bion's name for an emotional experience that consists in discovering coherence. Its meaning is in the relation among selected facts must not be considered logical," writes Bion in "A Theory of Thinking" (1961). The selected fact ties together or transforms the narrative story into a psychoanalytic account.

References

Bion, W. R.(1961) "A Theory of Thinking" *The International Journal of Psycho-Analysis*, 43, 306–10.

Grotstein, J. S. (2007). A beam of intense darkness: Wilfred Bion's legacy to psychoanalysis. Karnac Books London.

Williams. P. (2010) Invasive Objects: Minds under Siege Routledge London.

Index

For Product Safety Concerns and Information please contact our EU
representative GPSR@taylorandfrancis.com
Taylor & Francis Verlag GmbH, Kaufingerstraße 24, 80331 München, Germany